Cardiopulmonary Anatomy and Physiology

L. R. Matthews, RRT(A), MA
Respiratory Therapy Program
University College of the Cariboo
Kamloops, British Columbia
Canada

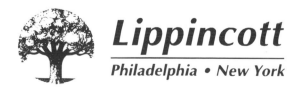

Lippincott
Philadelphia • New York

Associate Editor: Kathleen P. Lyons
Developmental Editor: Crystal G. Norris
Editorial Assistant: Stephanie R. Harold
Production Editor: Virginia Barishek
Production Manager: Janet Greenwood
Production: Colophon
Cover Design: Jerry Cable
Indexer: Beta Computer Indexing
Compositor: Maryland Composition Company
Cover Printer: Lehigh Press Lithographers
Printer/Binder: R.R. Donnelley & Sons Company/Crawfordsville

Library of Congress Cataloging-in-Publication Data

Matthews, L. R. (Les R.)
    Cardiopulmonary anatomy and physiology/L.R. Matthews.
        p.   cm.
    Includes bibliographical references and index.
    ISBN 0-397-54954-7
    1. Cardiopulmonary system—Physiology.   2. Cardiopulmonary system—
Anatomy.   I. Title.
        [DNLM: 1. Respiratory Mechanics—physiology.   2. Lung—physiology.
    3. Heart—physiology.   WF 102 M439c   1996]
    QP121.M378   1996
    612.2—dc20
    DNLM/DLC
    for Library of Congress   96-4884
                                                                       CIP

The material contained in this volume was submitted as previously unpublished material, except in the instances in which credit has been given to the source from which some of the illustrative material was derived.

Any procedure or practice described in this book should be applied by the health-care practitioner under appropriate supervision in accordance with professional standards of care used with regard to the unique circumstances that apply in each practice situation. Care has been taken to confirm the accuracy of information presented and to describe generally accepted practices. However, the authors, editors, and publisher cannot accept any responsibility for errors or omissions or for any consequences from application of the information in this book and make no warranty, express or implied, with respect to the contents of the book.

The authors and publisher have exerted every effort to ensure that drug selection and dosage set forth in this text are in accordance with current recommendations and practice at the time of publication. However, in view of ongoing research, changes in government regulations, and the constant flow of information relating to drug therapy and drug reactions, the reader is urged to check the package insert for each drug for any change in indications and dosage and for added warnings and precautions. This is particularly important when the recommended agent is a new or infrequently employed drug.

Materials appearing in this book prepared by individuals as part of their official duties as U.S. Government employees are not covered by the above-mentioned copyright.

9   8   7   6   5   4   3   2   1

PREFACE

Cardiopulmonary Anatomy and Physiology is designed to teach readers the fundamentals needed to understand the physiology of ventilation—from the normal, automatic process we know as breathing, or spontaneous ventilation, to machine-assisted ventilation. In order to understand this intricate process, the reader must first become familiar with gas exchange, hemodynamics, pharmacology, and pathophysiology.

Because the focus of this text is applied physiology, a prerequisite knowledge of basic anatomy is assumed. Chapter 1 provides a quick review of respiratory anatomy and the basic muscle physiology needed to understand spontaneous ventilation. Also, whenever relevant, chapters begin with the pertinent anatomy for the reader's ease of reference.

Chapters 2 through 5 are an overview of ventilation in process. Areas of focus include the work of breathing, particularly as it relates to compliance and resistance, two ever-present forces to be overcome in order to effect spontaneous ventilation; control of ventilatory patterns; and lung volumes and capacities and their interrelationship to gas flow.

Chapter 6 begins the discussion of pulmonary gas exchange. The five chapters that follow are designed to be read as a unit, which is organized to parallel the oxygen molecule's path through the cardiopulmonary system. Although this organizational strategy provides a useful unifying structure, it sometimes demands that I jump ahead of myself in explaining various concepts. I have done my best to keep this to a minimum. In cases where it was necessary to reference a term prior to its formal introduction in the text, the reader should refer to the glossary, which includes detailed explanations of key words and concepts. Readers who are more comfortable with a more traditional approach to the subject matter are invited to read Chapters 7 through 11 in the following order: (1) The Heart, (2) Circulation, (3) Gas Transport and the Red Blood Cell, (4) Pulmonary Circulation, and (5) Ventilation–Perfusion Relationships.

Chapters 12 (Fluids and Electrolyte Balance), 13 (Acid-Base Balance), and 14 (Blood Gases) detail the physiology of maintaining the body's internal environment (homeostasis) in terms of the cardiopulmonary system and the processes that support the functioning of that system. Chapter 15 (Pulmonary Defense Mechanisms) also addresses the problem of maintaining systemic homeostasis, from the standpoint of preserving the respiratory system from being breached by invasive organisms or particulate matter. This chapter resumes the anatomical train of thought by concentrating on the specifics of the respiratory lining and its role in protecting the integrity of the respiratory system.

Chapters are organized so that the reader has a clear idea from the onset which concepts are to be reviewed in each chapter. In addition to the chapter outline at the start of each chapter, which introduces the reader to what is to be covered, objectives have also been included with each chapter. The objectives define what the reader is expected to be able to do once the chapter is completed.

Each chapter concludes with a number of review questions which test the reader's knowledge of the concepts that have been learned by asking the reader to apply these concepts to problems. Answers to these questions can be found at the back of the book.

Scattered throughout the first few chapters of the book are "clinical applications" displays, which serve to reinforce the text's emphasis on the need for the reader to obtain a host of practicable skills. The clinical applications will address helpful assessment techniques and/or hints on how to interpret the various measurements of cardiopulmonary function.

Three additional features that the reader may find helpful are:

1. A list of abbreviations and symbols: This list is not limited to those items found in the text proper. It includes abbreviations and symbols that might be mentioned in any respiratory therapist's conversation.
2. Glossary: This section includes reiterated definitions of terms that were first introduced in boldface in the text. Generally speaking, this glossary is limited to nonanatomical terms. Anatomical terms have been set in italics within the text.
3. Lists of gas symbols and laws: These brief sections reiterate various gas laws and how they apply to ventilation.

I trust that the introduction of these features will reinforce the foundations of the reader's background knowledge, or expand upon it, without detracting from the text's primary focus on applied physiology.

Acknowledgments

I would like to acknowledge my wife Leslie for her long hours spent at the keyboard entering my manuscript. Without her help and dedication I would not have completed this project. Crystal Norris, my developmental editor, was extremely helpful and patient. I would also like to thank Sandy Van Mol, our department secretary, for all her help and support. Bryan Daly also helped me with illustrations, spending his time and saving mine. Cliff Seville and Dr. Chris Soder took time out of their busy schedules to review my manuscript and provided valuable feedback. John Andruschak remains the close friend, providing moral support through thick and thin.

L. R. Matthews, RRT(A), MA

CONTENTS

12
Fluids and Electrolyte Balance 239

13
Acid–Base Balance 257

To my wife, Leslie, and my children, James and Jessica. Their patience, love, and understanding made this book possible.

1

BASIC ANATOMY AND PHYSIOLOGY REVISITED

OBJECTIVES

1. Review the anatomy of the respiratory system, including the airways and the lungs (including the lobes, segments, and alveoli).

2. Review the anatomy of the chest, describing the landmarks of its anterior and posterior portions.

3. Describe how the thorax changes volume during inspiration and expiration.

4. Contrast and compare the pump-handle and bucket-handle effects.

5. Review the muscles of the thorax, abdomen, and upper limbs, and discuss their respective roles in the process of ventilation.

6. Discuss the physiology of skeletal muscle contraction.

Matthews LR: CARDIOPULMONARY ANATOMY AND PHYSIOLOGY. © 1996 Lippincott–Raven Publishers.

7. Describe skeletal muscle function in terms of strength, power, and endurance.

8. Explain energy production in terms of the phosphagen system, the glycogen-lactic acid system, and the aerobic system.

9. Describe the various energy sources used in muscle contraction.

The purpose of this chapter is twofold: to give readers an overall appreciation for breathing as a dynamic physiological function while reacquainting them with the basic anatomy and physiology that support normal respiration.

Breathing, or **spontaneous ventilation,** is defined as the process by which oxygen (O_2) from the external environment is taken into the lungs and exchanged for carbon dioxide (CO_2), which is then released into the environment. This gas exchange takes place within the respiratory tract, a system of connecting tubes, or *airways*, that progressively increases up to 70–100 square meters in area and volume to accommodate the demands of gas exchange.

Our discussion of how the process of spontaneous ventilation unfolds begins with a review of the airways and the lungs and then moves on to a macroscopic view of the chest. This approach of familiarizing the reader with the external landmarks and important points of reference provides a solid foundation for future applications of theory. Given that respiratory therapists routinely perform chest assessments, it is only reasonable that they be schooled in clinically relevant techniques for doing so as soon as possible.

Once the reader is familiar with the outside of the chest, we move deeper beneath the surface to explore the underlying skeletal structures and the muscles with which they work in tandem to achieve spontaneous ventilation. The chapter closes with a discussion of muscle physiology and the muscular work of normal breathing. With all of these fundamentals firmly in hand, the reader will be well equipped to move on to Chapter 2, which provides an overview of the dynamic process of spontaneous ventilation.

▼ ANATOMY

The Airways

Air from the outside environment enters the respiratory tract through the *oral* and *nasal cavities* and eventually winds its way through a series of connecting airways that end at the *alveolar ducts* and *alveolar sacs*.

The respiratory tract is divided into the upper and lower airways. The upper airway extends from the *anterior nares* to the *true vocal cords*. The lower airway extends from the true vocal cords (*false cords* are the *vestibular folds*) down to the *alveoli*, the lungs' gas exchange units.

The Upper Airways

The upper airway treats inspired air—either by heating or cooling it to 37° C, filtering it, and humidifying it—as it is conducted into the lower airway. The upper airway also provides for olfaction, the sense of smell. Without the upper airway, phonation, or sound production, would have a "nasal" quality.

The Nose

The *nose* is one of the two points of entry for air into the respiratory tract (the mouth is the other). It is composed of rigid bone and pliable fibrinous, cartilaginous, and epithelial tissues. It can be divided into four areas:

1. The external opening, or *nostrils*, bordered by the *ala nasae* (literally "wings of the nose")
2. The vestibular area just inside each nostril
3. The olfactory area
4. Nasal cavity

The nostrils, which include the *external* and *internal nares*, are made up of a pliable combination of fibrous tissue. This tissue serves the dual purpose of (1) maintaining the passages in their naturally open state and (2) allowing for dilation (achieved by nasal flaring) in an attempt to reduce airway resistance and reduce the work of breathing (see Chapter 3, "Control of Ventilation and Ventilatory Patterns," for a discussion of airway resistance).

The *vestibular area* is just inside each nostril and in the forefront of the *nasal fossa*, which extends into the *nasopharynx*. It should be kept in mind that this entire region is divided in two by the *septal cartilage*. This area is lined with *stratified squamous epithelium* (tissue made up of several layers of cells arranged in bricklike layers) and contains *cilia*, or nasal hairs, which provide an initial filtering system to remove large particles from the inspired air (see Chapter 14, "Pulmonary Defense Mechanisms," for information on the nose's role in defending the lungs from invasion by infectious organisms and particles).

Each nasal fossa, which extends from the vestibule to the nasopharynx, is outfitted with olfactory epithelium for the sense of smell. It contains three bony prominences: the superior, middle, and inner conchae, or *turbinates* (Figure 1-1). These structures increase the total surface area of the cavity, and are lined with ciliated pseudostratified columnar epithelium. This is important because it houses the mucus-producing goblet cells (see Chapter 15, "Pulmonary Defense Mechanisms").

The turbinates create three distinctive passageways known as *meati*, which heat, humidify, and filter inspired gases. By the time the inspired gas enters the nasopharynx, it is approximately 80% humidified. (The nasal mucosa actually gives up to 1 liter of water to inspired air per day.) This area is also efficient at filtering out foreign particles larger than 5 microns in diameter (see Chapter 15). The inconsistent nature of this passageway is of interest because it causes turbulent flow to increase contact between the gas and the mucous membrane.

Surrounding the nasal cavity are the *sinuses*. Although they aid in reducing the weight of the skull and take part in resonance, their definitive function has not been uncovered. There are four groups of *paranasal sinuses*:

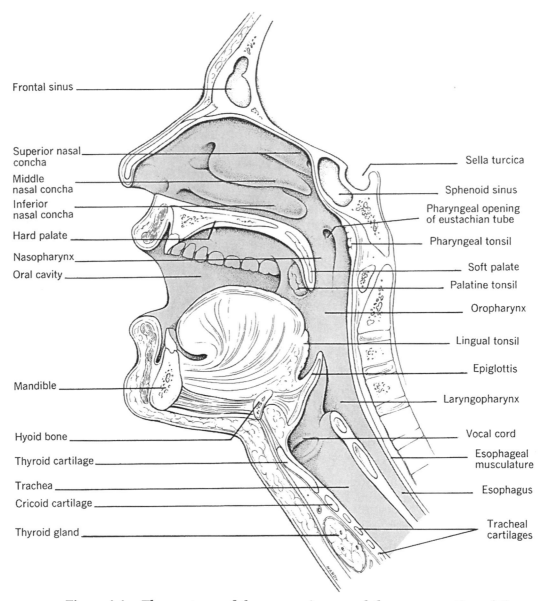

Figure 1-1.   The anatomy of the upper airway and the upper portion of the lower airway. (Chaffee, E.E. and Lytle, I.M., Basic Physiology and Anatomy, 4th ed. Philadelphia: J.B. Lippincott, 1980, with permission.)

1. Frontal
2. Maxillary
3. Sphenoidal
4. Ethmoidal

These sinuses are lined with *pseudostratified ciliated columnar epithelium* and produce mucus, which constantly drains into the *nasal meati*. Any condition or procedure that impedes this drainage can cause an extremely uncomfortable condition known as sinusitis.

The Pharynx

The *pharynx* extends from the posterior turbinates to the larynx, or esophagus. It is approximately 13 cm in length and serves as a common passageway for respiratory gases, nutrition, and fluid. The pharynx can be subdivided into the *nasopharynx*, *oropharynx*, and *laryngopharynx*.

The Nasopharynx.   The *nasopharynx* extends from the posterior turbinates to the *uvula*, the small dollop of tissue that hangs from the soft palate at the back of the throat. It, too, is lined with pseudostratified ciliated columnar epithelium. The eustachian tubes enter this region. Both the *pharyngeal* and *adenoid tonsils* are also located in this area.

The Oropharynx.   The *oropharynx* begins at the tip of the uvula and ends at the tip of the epiglottis. This area is lined with stratified squamous epithelium and houses the *lingual* and *palatine tonsils*.

The Laryngopharynx.   The *laryngopharynx*, also known as the *hypopharynx*, begins at the tip of the epiglottis and ends at the bifurcation between the larynx and the esophagus.

The Lower Airways

The Larynx

The *larynx*, which is lined with stratified squamous epithelium, is often referred to as the "voice box." In women the internal dimension of the larynx is approximately 8 mm wide and 16 mm deep. In men it is approximately 12 mm wide and 24 mm deep. Innervation of the larynx is vagal and occurs through the recurrent *laryngeal nerve*. Inappropriate stimulation of the larynx can result in laryngospasm, with devastating results from a lack of pulmonary ventilation.

Internal and external muscles make this a very active and important part of the respiratory system. Sound production and airway protection are its primary functions. An x-ray will show that the superior surface of the larynx normally sits between the third and sixth cervical vertebrae (C_3 and C_6).

Laryngeal Cartilages.   There are three unpaired cartilages (the *thyroid* and *cricoid cartilages* and the *epiglottis*) and three paired cartilages (the *arytenoid*, *corniculate*, and *cuneiform*) (Figure 1-2).

The epiglottis, a thin, lidlike structure that keeps the airway isolated from

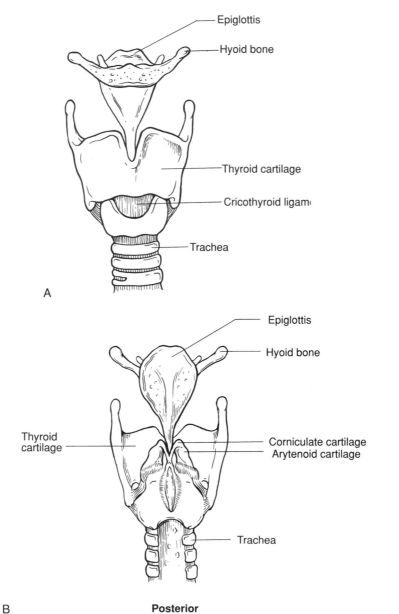

Figure 1-2.   The larynx: (a) anterior view, (b) posterior view, and (c) cross-sectional view.

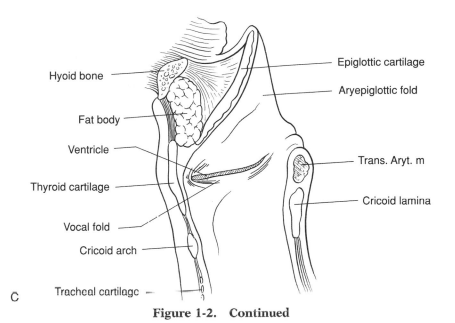

Hyoid bone

Fat body

Ventricle

Thyroid cartilage

Vocal fold

Cricoid arch

C   Tracheal cartilage

Epiglottic cartilage

Aryepiglottic fold

Trans. Aryt. m

Cricoid lamina

Figure 1-2.   Continued

the esophagus, plays an important role in the swallowing mechanism. The thyroid cartilage, more commonly known as the "Adam's apple," is the largest laryngeal cartilage. The cricoid cartilage, which lies anterior to the esophagus, can help prevent gastric reflux when pressure is exerted on it.

Laryngeal Ligaments.   Laryngeal ligaments are both intrinsic and extrinsic. The *extrinsic ligaments* connect the thyroid cartilage and the epiglottis with the horseshoe-shaped *hyoid* bone, at the base of the tongue. They also connect the cricoid cartilage with the trachea. The *intrinsic ligaments* are responsible for the connections between cartilages of the larynx. The *cricothyroid ligament* is of particular importance because it is the site of emergency tracheostomies (cricothyrotomies). Because of its proximity to the vocal cords and related concerns about long-term laryngeal or vocal cord ramifications, the cricothyroid ligament is never selected as the site for elective tracheostomies (Figure 1-3).

The Trachea
The *trachea* is a flexible tube that begins at the larynx and ends at the bifurcation of the right and left mainstem *bronchi*, the two main passageways leading directly into the lungs. Lying directly in front of the esophagus, it is approximately 10–13 cm in length and 2.5 cm in diameter. The walls contain 16–20 U-shaped tracheal cartilages. The U is open posteriorly. The opening is connected by smooth muscle and connective tissue. The wall of the trachea contains ciliated pseudostratified columnar epithelium, which contains both mucosal and submucosal glands for mucus production (see Chapter 15 for a detailed description of the airway mucosa).

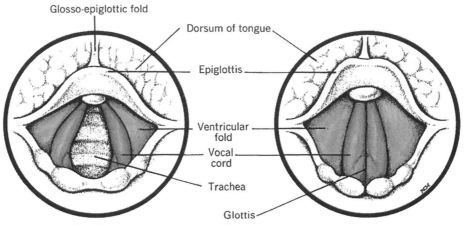

Figure 1-3.   The larynx as seen through a laryngoscope. (Chaffee, E.E. and Lytle, I.M., Basic Physiology and Anatomy, 4th ed. Philadelphia: J.B. Lippincott, 1980, with permission.)

The Tracheobronchial Tree

Each lung is connected to the trachea via its respective mainstem bronchus. The *carina* is the ridge at the lower end of the trachea that separates it into the left and right mainstem bronchi. The right mainstem bronchus comes off the trachea at 20–30° from midline then subdivides. The left mainstem bronchus comes off the trachea 40–60° from midline.

Each of the mainstem bronchi further subdivides into successively smaller airways, or *bronchioles*, for up to 23–27 *generations*, or successive subdivisions (Figure 1-4). The penultimate subdivision of a bronchiole is referred to as the *terminal bronchiole* and leads to the *respiratory bronchiole*. The respiratory bronchioles are important because they lead into the *alveolar ducts*, which communicate with the *alveoli*, the site where O_2 and CO_2 are exchanged within the lung. There are approximately 300,000,000 of these gas exchange units in the human lung (Figure 1-5).

The Lungs

The lungs, the primary organs of respiration, are situated in the pleural cavity of the thorax. Each lung is connected to the trachea by a bifurcation of the mainstem bronchus and rests its base on the diaphragm.

The right lung has three lobes: the upper (superior), middle, and lower (inferior) lobes. These are each subdivided into segments. The right superior lobe contains three segments (*apical, posterior*, and *anterior*). The right middle lobe contains two segments (*lateral* and *medial*). The right inferior lobe contains five segments (*superior, medial basal, anterior basal, lateral basal*, and *posterior basal*).

The left lung differs from the right in two important respects: it has two, not three, lobes (superior and inferior) and an indentation (cardiac depression)

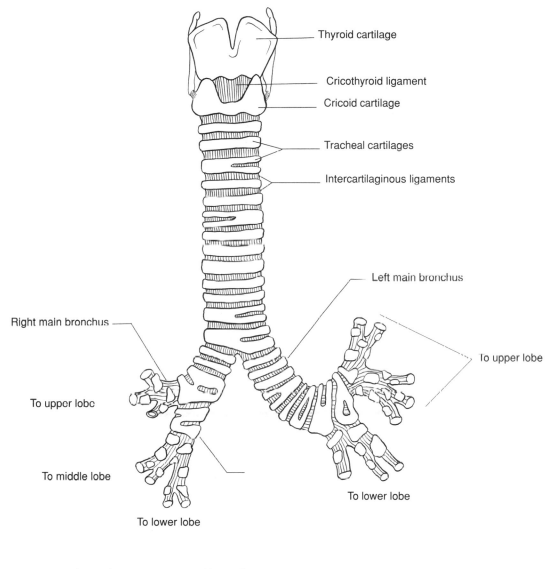

A   Intrapulmonary   Extrapulmonary   Intrapulmonary

Figure 1-4.   (a) The trachea and its subsequent subdivisions (generations) are depicted. (b) The generations in the human airway and how they correspond to the structures in the lung already mentioned. The conducting airways comprise the first 16 generations; the last seven generations correspond to the respiratory zone. (B adapted from: Weibel, E.R., Morphometry of the Human Lung. New York: Springer-Verlag, 1962, with permission.)

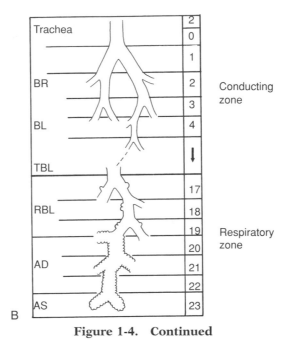

Figure 1-4.   Continued

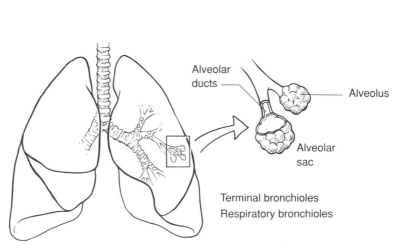

Figure 1-5.   Oxygen and carbon dioxide are exchanged in the lungs' estimated 300,000,000 alveoli.

to accommodate normal placement of the heart. The left superior lobe contains four segments (*apical posterior, anterior, superior lingular*, and *inferior lingular*). The left inferior lobe divides into four segments (*superior, anteromedial basal, lateral basal*, and *posterior basal*).

A frontal view of the lungs clearly shows the division between lobes on both the right and left sides. The division between the right superior and middle lobes is known as the *horizontal fissure*. The division between the middle and inferior lobes is known as the *oblique fissure*. On the left side, the upper and lower lobe fissure is known as the *oblique fissure*. Segmental differentiation of the lung is not externally visible (Figure 1-6).

Anatomy of the Chest

The chest, or *thorax*, is that part of the body that lies between the base of the neck and the muscular sheath of the diaphragm. It is actually the bony cage that houses and protects the cardiopulmonary organs. The look and feel of the

---

Clinical Applications Box 1-1   Clinical Applications: Assessing Chest Expansion

The chest expands in a symmetrical fashion during maximal inspiration. This expansion can be assessed by external examination techniques. One method is to ask the patient to exhale maximally. The examiner's hands are then gently placed on the patient's back, opened, and moved down until the thumbs meet at the midvertebral line. The patient is then instructed to take a deep breath. The examiner's thumbs should separate an equal distance from the spine so that there is a total of 6–10 cm (2–4 inches) between them.

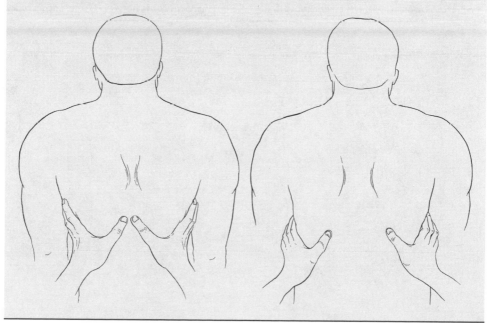

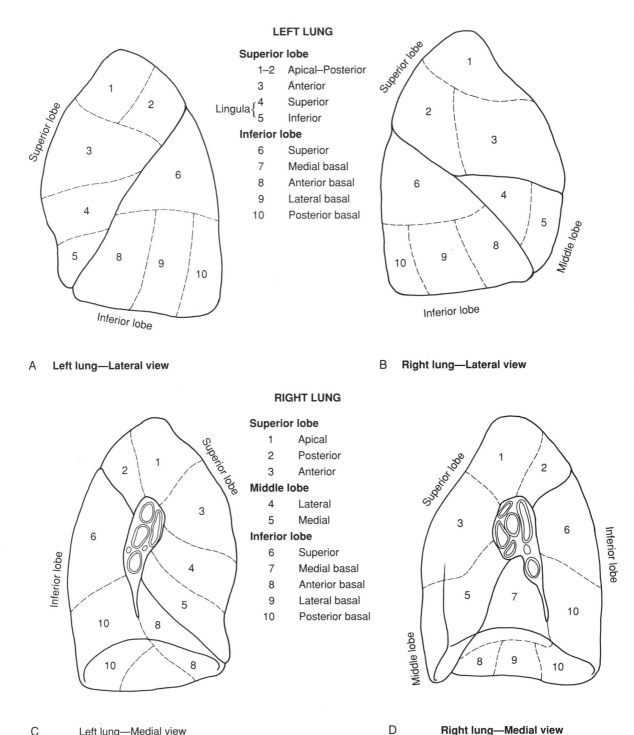

LEFT LUNG

Superior lobe
1–2   Apical–Posterior
3   Anterior
Lingula { 4   Superior
5   Inferior
Inferior lobe
6   Superior
7   Medial basal
8   Anterior basal
9   Lateral basal
10   Posterior basal

A   **Left lung—Lateral view**

B   **Right lung—Lateral view**

RIGHT LUNG

Superior lobe
1   Apical
2   Posterior
3   Anterior
Middle lobe
4   Lateral
5   Medial
Inferior lobe
6   Superior
7   Medial basal
8   Anterior basal
9   Lateral basal
10   Posterior basal

C   Left lung—Medial view

D   **Right lung—Medial view**

Figure 1-6. The segmental breakdown of the lungs.

chest can give the respiratory therapist valuable clues as to how the work of spontaneous ventilation is being performed.

Chest assessment involves a series of steps: mensuration (the taking of measurements), palpation, and percussion (see Clinical Applications Box 1-1 for a guide to examining the patient with respiratory difficulties). Although it is beyond the scope of this text to describe each phase of chest assessment in detail, it is certainly within its scope to introduce the landmarks and imaginary lines that segment the chest into discrete sections. After all, these topographical markers convey to the respiratory therapist a great deal of information about the underlying soundness or dysfunction of the anatomical structures involved in spontaneous ventilation.

Chest Divisions

The anterior, lateral, and posterior views of the chest depicted in Figure 1-7 give the respiratory therapist three different perspectives and thus three separate opportunities to detect any potential abnormalities.

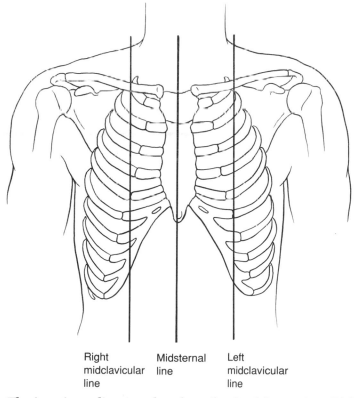

Right
midclavicular
line

Midsternal
line

Left
midclavicular
line

A

Figure 1-7.   The imaginary lines used to describe the (a) anterior, (b) lateral, and (c) posterior views of the chest wall.

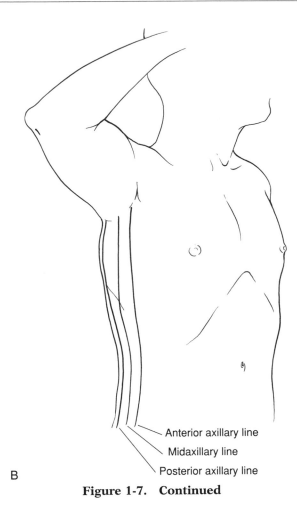

B

Figure 1-7.   Continued

Anterior Chest

The anterior chest is divided into two halves by the *midsternal line*. Each half is further subdivided into two parts by a parallel *midclavicular line* (Figure 1-7a).

The *sternum*, or breastbone, forms the anterior surface of the chest. The *sternal notch* (sometimes known as the suprasternal notch) is located on the superior surface of the *manubrium*, which articulates with the *clavicle* and the first pair of costal cartilages. The point at which the manubrium joins to the body of the sternum (gladiolus) is called the angle of Louis or, more simply, the *sternal angle* (Figure 1-8a).

The second to the seventh ribs on each side are directly attached to the sternum by their respective cartilages. [The attachment of the second set of ribs actually falls directly in line with the sternal angle (Figure 1-8a).] In contrast, the eighth, ninth, and tenth ribs on each side share a common cartilagi-

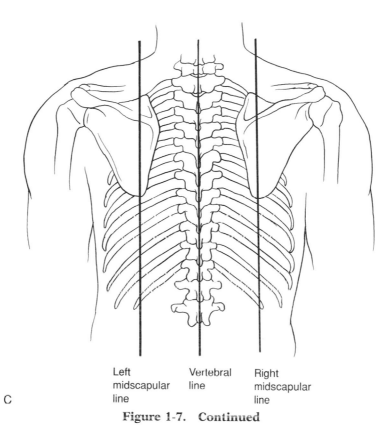

Left   Vertebral   Right
midscapular   line   midscapular
line   line

C

Figure 1-7.   Continued

nous connection with the sternum. The 11th and 12th ribs are free floating, and as such articulate only with the spine.

Generally, the lungs do not extend below the sixth or seventh rib anteriorly. If they do, it is a sign of hyperinflation. See Figure 1-8a for the lungs' relative positions within the thoracic cavity from both the anterior and posterior perspectives.

There are two points of articulation between each rib and its corresponding vertebra: one is between the head of the rib and the body of the vertebra; the other is between the *costal tubercle* and the *vertebral transverse process* (Figure 1-8b).

Posterior Chest

Posteriorly, the chest is divided into two halves by the *midvertebral line* (Figure 1-7c). Running parallel on either side of this imaginary median are the left and right *midscapular lines*.

The posterior view of the chest allows for visualization of how the ribs articulate with the vertebrae. At the base of the neck lies the most prominent spinous process, C_7; the first set of ribs articulates with the thoracic cage at T_1, the spinous process immediately below C_7. These particular spinal column

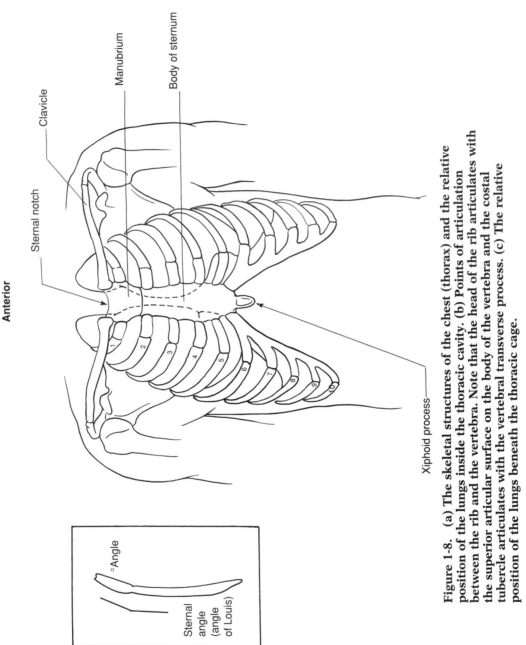

Figure 1-8. (a) The skeletal structures of the chest (thorax) and the relative position of the lungs inside the thoracic cavity. (b) Points of articulation between the rib and the vertebra. Note that the head of the rib articulates with the superior articular surface on the body of the vertebra and the costal tubercle articulates with the vertebral transverse process. (c) The relative position of the lungs beneath the thoracic cage.

Posterior

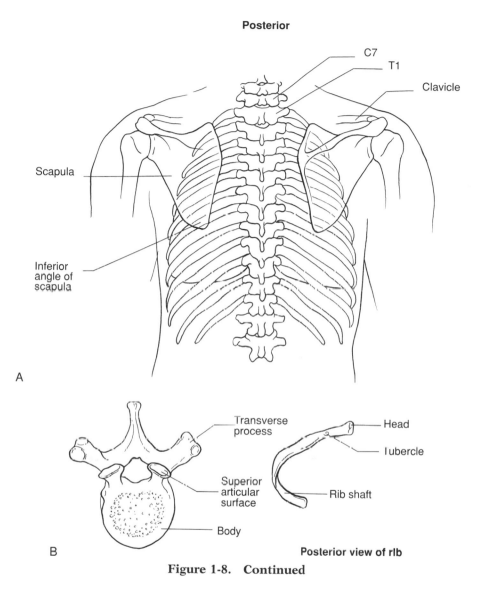

B

Posterior view of rib

Figure 1-8.   Continued

landmarks provide points of reference that allow the respiratory therapist to locate for assessment of the lung fissures, the carina, and the diaphragm (Figure 1-8c) (see Clinical Applications Box 1-2 for a review of a standardized method of identifying these vertebral sites).

Muscles of Ventilation

The muscles of the chest work together to support the rigid bony thorax containing the lungs and to inhibit the lungs' natural tendency to collapse. These

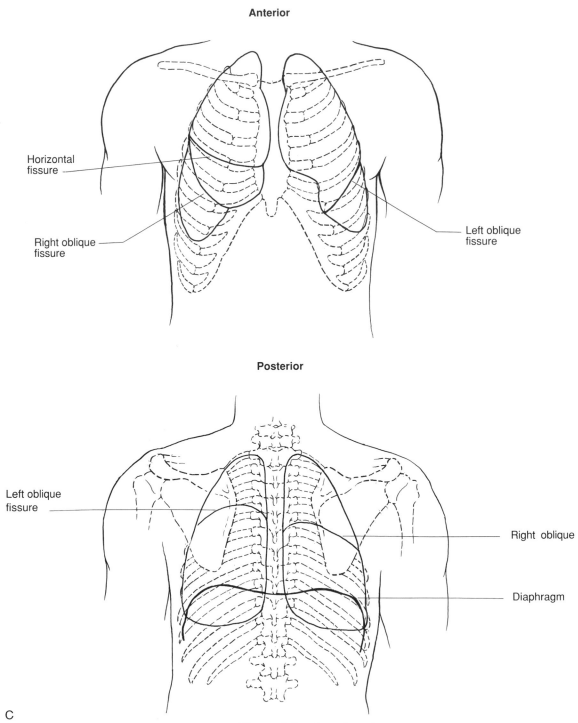

Anterior

Horizontal
fissure

Right oblique
fissure

Left oblique
fissure

Posterior

Left oblique
fissure

Right oblique

Diaphragm

C

Figure 1-8.   Continued

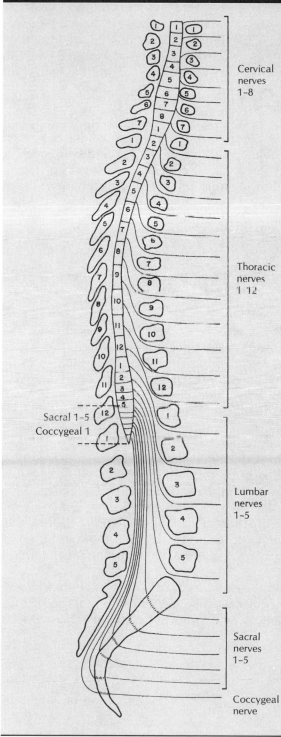

Cervical
nerves
1–8

Thoracic
nerves
1–12

Sacral 1–5
Coccygeal 1

Lumbar
nerves
1–5

Sacral
nerves
1–5

Coccygeal
nerve

The spinal column is segmented into five distinct sections, or curves. Each curve has a set number of vertebrae, or spiny processes: cervical, 7; thoracic, 12; lumbar, 5; sacral, 5 bones fused into 1; coccyx, 4 bones fused to form 1. Identifying these bones is standardized so that the spinal region is listed, followed by the number of the vertebra being examined. For example, T_1 refers to the first thoracic vertebra. (Figure from: Barr, M.L. and Kiernan, J.A., The Human Nervous System: An Anatomical Viewpoint, 5th ed. Philadelphia: J.B. Lippincott, 1993, with permission.)

muscles of ventilation, which are classified as either inspiratory or expiratory, pump the chest to move a volume of air into and out of the lungs in much the same fashion that a water pump moves water from an underground well into a bucket (see Clinical Application Box 1-3 for an explanation of the bucket-handle and pump-handle effects).

Inspiratory Muscles

Inspiratory muscles are used to elevate the chest cage and force the diaphragm downward to increase thoracic volume (Figure 1-9a). These muscles, led by the diaphragm and the external intercostals, consume almost all of the O_2 needed to fuel ventilation. The following muscles provide this function (Figure 1-9):

1. Diaphragm (a combination of muscles and fibrous septum)[*]
2. External intercostals[*]
3. Sternocleidomastoid
4. Anterior serratus
5. Scalene (posterior, anterior, medial)
6. Pectoralis minor and major

The *diaphragm* (Figure 1-9b) is actually composed of two muscles that are connected medially by a fibrous septum. This dome-shaped arc of muscle consists of three leaflets (right, center, and left), which are tendinous in the center and wrapped in an outer layer of muscle. These muscles can be described by their points of origin as sternal, costal, or lumbar.

The moveable musculature of the diaphragm, which separates the thoracic and abdominal cavities, has a significant impact on thoracic volume. On its own, it is capable only of contracting and moving downward to increase the vertical dimension of the thorax during inspiration. During quiet respiration, this contraction typically measures 1–2 cm. In order to effect upward movement of the diaphragm, the abdominal muscles must be contracted to push abdominal contents upward.

Although the muscles of the diaphragm normally function as a unit, they are innervated by two separate *phrenic nerves*, the left and the right. Damage to one nerve affects only that half of the diaphragm (hemidiaphragm) that it innervates.

The *external intercostals* (Figure 1-9c and d) are instrumental in achieving the bucket-handle effect: they contract during inspiration to pull the ribs forward and upward, thus increasing thoracic volume (the lateral and anteroposterior diameters).

Accessory Muscles of Ventilation

When the respiratory system is pushed to the limits of its reserve, *accessory muscle* recruitment becomes necessary. Clinical identification of activity of

---

[*] These muscles are used during normal, quiet breathing.

Clinical Applications Box 1-3   Skeletal Mechanics of Breathing

The following two well-known effects explain how the ribs move to accommodate changes in thoracic volume. Their names are adapted from the water-pump analogy mentioned previously.

Pump-Handle Effect

The upper part of the thorax is conical and slopes forward. The ribs, which attach to the sternum below their points of articulation with the spine, can lift the sternum to increase the anterior-posterior (A-P) diameter of the chest. Because the lower ribs are not directly aligned with the sternum, they contribute very little to this increased A-P diameter. During expiration this entire process occurs in reverse, resulting in a decreased A-P diameter.

Bucket-Handle Effect

All of the moveable ribs from the second to the tenth articulate with the spine and the sternum. (Remember, the free-floating 11th and 12th sets of ribs do not attach to the sternum.) Because the center of each set of moveable ribs lies lower than their points of articulation with the spine and the sternum, the ribs are lifted upward during inspiration to accommodate an increase in lateral chest diameter. The reverse occurs during expiration, resulting in a decreased transverse diameter.

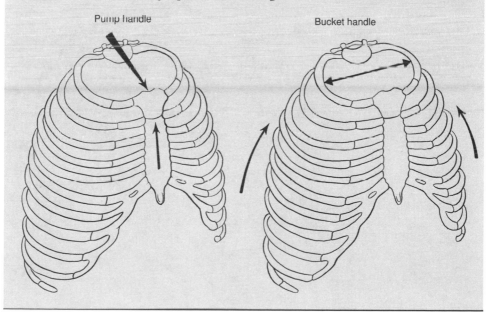

Pump handle   Bucket handle

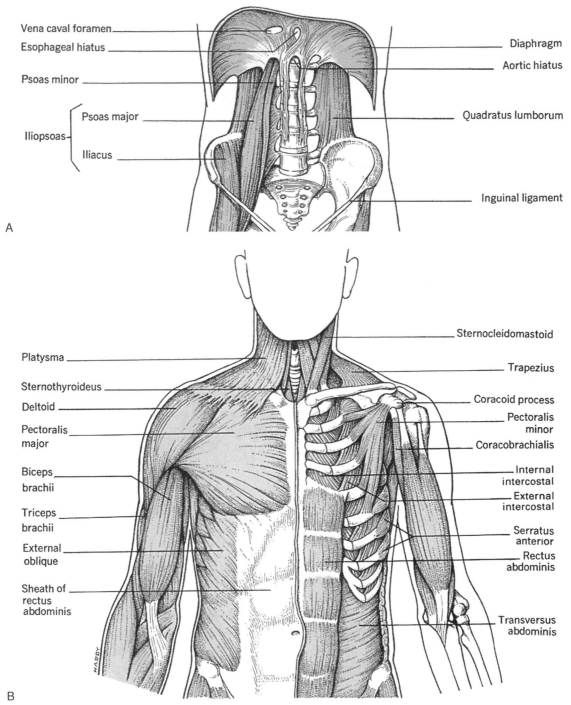

Figure 1-9.   (a) The muscles of inspiration. (b) The diaphragm is a dome of moveable musculature that separates the abdominal and thoracic cavities. (c) The expiratory muscles. (d) Accessory muscles of ventilation. (Chaffee, E.E. and Lytle, I.M., Basic Physiology and Anatomy, 4th ed. Philadelphia: J.B. Lippincott, 1980, with permission.)

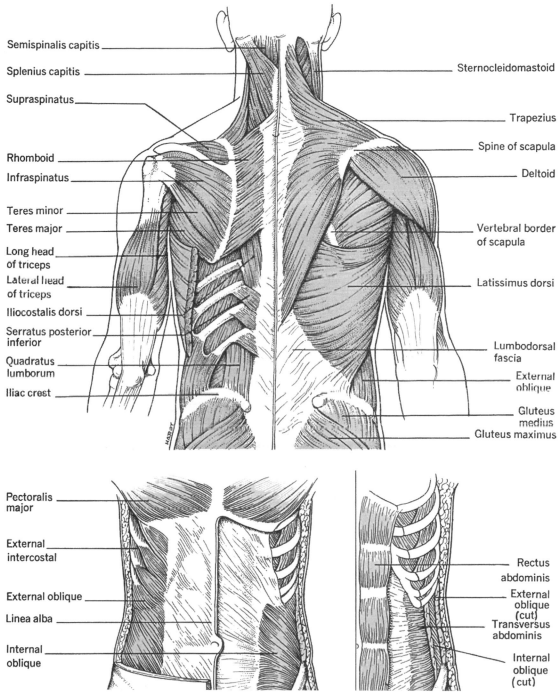

Semispinalis capitis

Splenius capitis

Supraspinatus

Rhomboid

Infraspinatus

Teres minor

Teres major

Long head of triceps

Lateral head of triceps

Iliocostalis dorsi

Serratus posterior inferior

Quadratus lumborum

Iliac crest

C

Sternocleidomastoid

Trapezius

Spine of scapula

Deltoid

Vertebral border of scapula

Latissimus dorsi

Lumbodorsal fascia

External oblique

Gluteus medius

Gluteus maximus

Pectoralis major

External intercostal

External oblique

Linea alba

Internal oblique

D

Rectus abdominis

External oblique (cut)

Transversus abdominis

Internal oblique (cut)

Figure 1-9. Continued

these muscle groups, which remain uninvolved during healthy ventilation, is important in recognizing chronic or impending ventilatory failure.

The *sternocleidomastoid* muscles (Figure 1-9c) push up on the sternum, also increasing thoracic volume, this time via the pump-handle effect. The *anterior serrati* (Figure 1-9b) are responsible for lifting ribs upward. The *scalene muscles*, three muscles on each side of the neck that extend from spinous processes C_3 through C_6 and down to the first or second rib (Figure 1-9a), lift the first two ribs upward.

The *pectoralis muscles* may be recruited to raise the ribs and sternum during stressful ventilation. In patients with emphysema, for example, leaning or anchoring the forearms on a table or other flat surface can allow for the use of the pectoralis muscles to further expand the chest when ventilatory reserves are low or nonexistent.

Expiratory Muscles

The collective purpose of the expiratory muscles is to decrease thoracic volume (which drives up intrapleural pressure) and thereby force gas out of the lungs quickly. Expiration is normally the function of the natural recoil of the lungs and as such requires no overt muscular exertion. However, when demands are placed on the respiratory system, the expiratory muscles must be recruited to reduce the expiratory time and thereby increase the number of breaths per minute.

The following muscles work in concert to achieve expiration when there is an increased demand for O_2 uptake and CO_2 removal (e.g., during stress, exercise, or disease) (Figure 1-9b, and d):

1. Rectus abdominus
2. Transversus abdominus
3. Internal obliques
4. External obliques
5. Internal intercostals

The *rectus abdominus* pulls down on the lower ribs while it compresses abdominal contents to push upward on the diaphragm. The *transversus abdominus* and the *internal and external obliques* are all capable of joining in to serve this same function (forced expiration). The *internal intercostals* pull ribs backward and down, decreasing thoracic volume.

The end result of skeletal and muscular coordination is shown in Figure 1-10, which depicts normal inspiration and expiration.

Ventilatory Muscle Failure

Loss of ventilatory muscle function results in death almost immediately. With such a loss, some form of mechanical intervention becomes necessary. Mouth-to-mouth (or mask) resuscitation, resuscitation bag and mask, or automatic mechanical ventilation may be necessary if the person is to survive. Even partial failure of ventilatory muscle function can have devastating results, so respiratory care practitioners must pay close attention to both maintenance and reha-

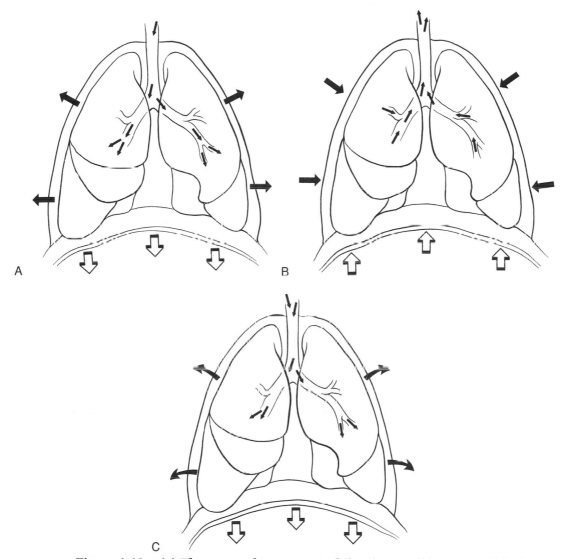

Figure 1-10.   (a) The outward movement of the chest wall is accomplished primarily by contraction of the intercostal muscles and the downward movement of the diaphragm. The resulting increased volume and decreased pressure cause air to flow into the lungs (inspiration). (b) The inward movement, or relaxation, of the chest wall is accomplished primarily by the intercostal muscles and the abdominal contents pushing the diaphragm back in place. This action decreases the volume and increases the pressure to force air out of the lung (expiration). (c) Gas moves into the lungs as the result of increased intrathoracic volume and decreased alveolar pressure.

bilitation of ventilatory muscle function. Disorders that have an impact on muscle function are too numerous to list in this context. However, they can be arranged in general categories to describe the causes of failure. Some of these disorders are listed as follows:

1. Central nervous system defects such as Ondine's curse, central sleep apnea, and drug overdose.
2. Neuronal defects such as spinal cord injuries and multiple sclerosis.
3. Neuromuscular function abnormalities such as myasthenia gravis and Guillain-Barré.
4. Muscular function abnormalities such as muscular dystrophy and myotonic dystrophy.
5. Thoracic cage abnormalities capable of affecting breathing efficiency by affecting the normal expansion process of the thorax include pectus carinatum, an abnormal anterior protrusion of the sternum; pectus excavatum, an abnormal depression of the sternum; kyphosis, an abnormal anteroposterior curvature of the spine; scoliosis, an abnormal lateral curvature of the spine; and kyphoscoliosis, the combined lateral and anteroposterior curvature of the spine.
6. Chest trauma. If the chest wall is relaxed, damaged, or unstable when the diaphragm contracts, instead of gas moving into the lungs from the mouth and nose, the chest wall simply collapses in response to the negative pressure generated inside the chest (Figure 1-11). When ribs are broken in more than one place, a flail chest may develop, as seen in Figure 1-11. Conversely, if the diaphragm is paralyzed during inspiration, it will move upward rather than downward when the intercostal muscles contract. In both cases, this ineffective action is referred to as *paradoxical movement*. *Respiratory alternans* is also paradoxical chest movement resulting from alternating diaphragm and intercostal breathing. It is usually a result of diaphragm muscle fatigue.

▼ A REVIEW OF MUSCLE PHYSIOLOGY

Before we delve into the sources of energy used to fuel the activity of the muscles of ventilation under normal circumstances, let us review the processes that take place on a cellular level to make this muscular movement possible.

The *sarcomere* is the contractile portion of a striated muscle fibril. Figure 1-12a shows a relaxed sarcomere with a normal resting membrane potential of the *sarcolemma* (surrounding membrane) and the *sarcoplasmic reticulum* (a network of T tubules found in muscle fibers). During this relaxed state, calcium ions are held in reservoirs located in the sarcoplasmic reticulum, and the cross-bridges between the thick, proteinaceous myosin and actin filaments are not yet engaged.

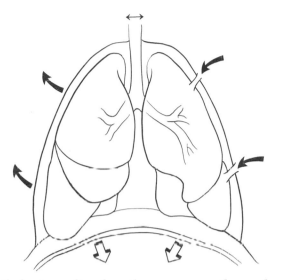

Figure 1-11.   Flail chest results when three or more ribs are broken in more than one place, which leads to the abnormal inward movement of the chest wall during inspiration.

The myosin filament is an incredibly complex strand of numerous myosin molecules. Each myosin molecule is a combination of six polypeptide chains. One end is folded into a globular protein mass commonly referred to as a myosin head; the other end is referred to as a tail. The myosin head is necessary for muscle contraction. It acts as an adenosine triphosphatase (ATPase) enzyme by cleaving the high-energy phosphate bonds of adenosine triphosphate (ATP) for the contractile proteins.

The actin filament is also an extremely complex strand composed of three components: actin, tropomyosin, and troponin. The actin and tropomyosin molecules are wound around each other like strands of twine. Troponin molecules are situated along the strands. Their high affinity for calcium implicates them in the initiation of the contractile process.

Stimulation of the muscle results in the depolarization of cellular membranes (sarcolemma), which in turn causes a release of calcium ions. This release of calcium stimulates a series of events that cause the hinged myosin bridges to repeatedly engage, tilt, and disengage from active sites on actin filaments. When actin filaments and attached Z bands are pulled inward among myosin filaments, the sarcomere contracts (Figure 1-12b).

Relaxation of the sarcomere, and thus the muscle, occurs when the action potential returns to normal. (Remember, an action potential results when the sodium-potassium pump creates an electrical potential from the inside to the outside of the cell membrane.) When this happens, calcium ions are returned

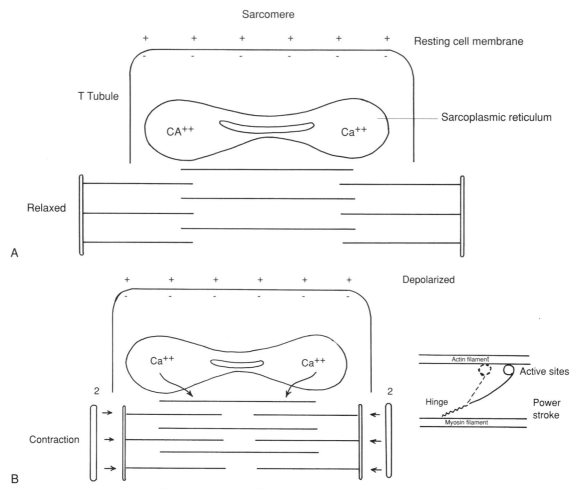

Figure 1-12. This schematic diagram shows the contraction and relaxation of skeletal muscle. Each and every breath requires that this process occur 900 times each hour, for a total of 20,000 times a day, or 8,000,000 times a year.

to binding sites in the sarcoplasmic reticulum and the muscle relaxes. Once the muscle achieves its resting potential, it is ready for another contraction (see Clinical Applications Box 1-4 for information on the graphing of muscular contraction in response to electrical stimulation).

Considerations in Muscle Function

Three aspects of skeletal muscle function dictate how well, or how efficiently, the muscle will work:

1. Strength
2. Power
3. Endurance

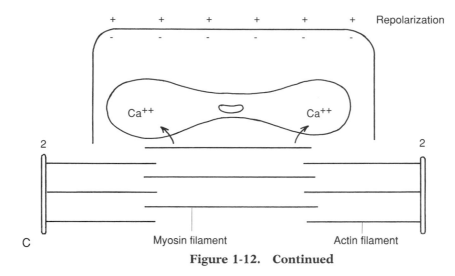

Figure 1-12. Continued

The contractile strength of a muscle, which is measured in kg/cm² of muscle cross-section, is determined primarily by its size. Hypertrophied (enlarged) muscle, in which the number of myofilaments is significantly greater than in the average cell, would be stronger than ordinary muscle. Muscle atrophy, on the other hand, can occur when the muscle either is not used or is used only for very weak contractions (as when the work of ventilation is taken over by a mechanical apparatus). Removal of nervous control (denervation) also results in muscle atrophy.

The power of a muscle contraction refers to its ability to work over a period of time. Work, in this case, is defined as the number of times a muscle can contract in one minute. This is measured in kg/m/minute, or the ability to move 1 kg 1 m in 60 seconds.

Endurance refers to the length of time a muscle can function before it becomes exhausted. The longer a muscle is able to function without becoming

---

Clinical Applications Box 1-4   Electromyographic Monitoring

An electromyogram (EMG) can be used to obtain a graphic representation of the muscle contraction. This is accomplished by inserting needle electrodes beneath the skin into the muscle. Electromyographic monitoring is a useful tool because it provides information on several physiological functions:

(a) central neural drive

(b) muscle dyscoordination

(c) muscle fatigue

In time, it may become a common and useful monitoring parameter for assessing ventilatory function.

fatigued, the more endurance it has. Hypertrophied muscle has more endurance than normal or underdeveloped muscle because it can distribute the same amount of work among a greater number of myofilaments. Even given the greater number of myofilaments, a muscle's endurance depends on its receiving adequate nutrition and O_2. The amount of glycogen (animal starch) stored in the muscle before physical exertion is the most important predictor of muscle endurance. Because glycogen can be formed from carbohydrate sources (glycogenesis), an individual on a high-carbohydrate diet will have far more glycogen stored in the muscles than someone on a high-fat diet and thus show substantial muscle endurance.

▼ ENERGY PRODUCTION FOR MUSCLE WORK

There are three systems that can be used to obtain the energy necessary for muscle contraction, each of which is based, respectively, on:

1. Phosphagen (ATP)
2. Glycogen-lactic acid
3. O_2 (the aerobic system)

Which system is activated depends on the conditions under which the muscles are required to work. The phosphagen system provides energy for very short-term energy expenditure (10–15 seconds). The glycogen-lactic acid system functions entirely in the absence of O_2. It produces lactic acid, resulting in lactic acidosis. This system can provide 30–40 seconds of maximum muscle activity.

The aerobic system uses O_2 continuously and is required for prolonged muscle use because it can supply a continuous source of energy for muscle function. Its metabolite is CO_2, a gas easily removed from the lung by breathing in greater depth and frequency, as required. (The ratio of exchange for O_2 and CO_2 is variable, from 0.7 while burning fat, to 0.8 while burning protein, to 1.0 while burning carbohydrates. The ratio of CO_2 produced, divided by O_2 consumed at a cellular level is known as the **respiratory quotient**. The ratio of CO_2 diffusing into the lung divided by the volume of O_2 diffusing into the blood is known as the **respiratory exchange ratio**.) The aerobic system is operational as long as available nutrients and O_2 last.

Energy Sources

ATP is the primary energy source for skeletal muscle contraction. This phosphate compound is energy rich and when split releases a burst of energy to power the interaction between actin and myosin. Myosin also acts as an enzyme to split ATP for the necessary release of energy.

Once the contractile process is complete, adenosine diphosphate (ADP) is immediately converted back to ATP. This occurs primarily when ADP reacts with phosphocreatine, another high-energy compound inside the sarcoplasm. Phosphocreatine exists in greater concentration than ATP but must channel its energy release through ATP to be used by the muscle.

$$ADP + phosphocreatine = ATP + creatine$$

ADP that is not converted to ATP through this process diffuses out of the myofibril (small fiber in muscle tissue) into the mitochondria (the cell's source of energy), where it is used in the citric acid cycle (Krebs cycle). The citric acid cycle is an oxidative process requiring a constant supply of O_2. At rest, or with moderate exercise, energy requirements can be met by this oxidative process in the mitochondria. However, during strenuous muscular activity such as a 100-meter dash, the available ATP is soon used up and the interaction of ADP and phosphocreatine becomes an important source of ATP.

The anaerobic breakdown of carbohydrates provides another source for muscle contraction. When O_2 is not available, a complex set of chemical reactions breaks down glycogen and glucose to produce pyruvic acid. This process produces relatively small amounts of ATP, but during times of stress this can provide an important source of energy to meet the increased demands of respiration. The availability of O_2 determines whether pyruvic acid becomes an important source of ATP production (Figure 1-13). Moderate exercise generally results in the oxidation of any circulating pyruvic acid. This oxidation converts

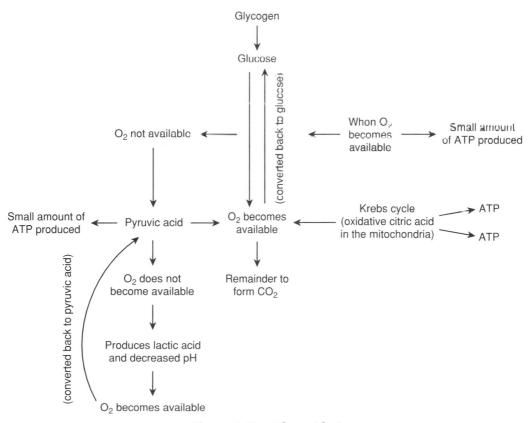

Figure 1-13. The oxidative process

some of the acid into CO_2 and water. The remainder is converted back into glycogen by the energy produced during this reaction. This balance of supply and demand is commonly referred to as a *steady state*.

If O_2 is not available in sufficient quantities, pyruvic acid is not effectively processed (Figure 1-13). Under these circumstances, pyruvic acid is converted back to lactic acid. If this O_2 debt is allowed to continue, a build-up of lactic acid may result in lactic acidosis and muscle fatigue. Lactic acidosis reduces muscle activity by directly reducing muscle irritability and contractility. If the O_2 balance is restored, lactic acid is converted back into pyruvic acid. Some is oxidized, which provides energy to convert the remainder back to glycogen and restore the phosphocreatine and ATP process.

The importance of the oxidative process within the mitochondria is easy to see. It replenishes the cellular energy stores, prevents the accumulation of lactic acid, and helps prevent the depletion of glycogen as a fuel supply.

Prolonged strong muscle contraction (such as that evidenced by patients with stiff lung from respiratory disease or trauma) leads to muscle fatigue. An insufficient supply of nutrients, O_2, and blood will also diminish muscle function. A balance of fluid and electrolytes is also important for effective muscle function. *Hypocalcemia* (decreased Ca^+ level), *hyponatremia* (decreased Na^+ level), and *hypokalemia* (decreased K^+ level) all result in reduced muscle contractility and a reduced capacity to meet the demands placed on the respiratory system (see Chapter 12, "Fluid and Electrolyte Balance").

▼ CONCLUSION

This chapter has reviewed basic respiratory anatomy from the upper to the lower airways. External landmarks associated with the internal organs have been identified for future implication in disease states. The most important area of focus of the chapter was the description of the thorax and its attached muscles as a pump that works constantly to move gas into and out of the lungs. Finally, muscle physiology was reviewed, showing the importance of muscle function underlying the act of breathing.

With a fundamental understanding of the mechanism of breathing, the reader will be able to proceed to a more comprehensive view of the respiratory system in health and disease.

❖ Review Questions

1. Paradoxical chest movement may result from
   i.   a paralyzed diaphragm.
   ii. a flail chest.
   iii. inspiration.
   iv. maximum expiration.
   v.   strenuous exercise.

   a. i, ii
   b. i, ii, iii
   c. ii, iii, iv
   d. iii, iv, v
   e. i, iii, iv

2. During quiet inspiration the diaphragm contracts approximately _____ cm.
   a. 1–2
   b. 2–6
   c. 3–5
   d. 4–8
   e. 10–15

3. Lifting the sternum and increasing the anterior-posterior diameter of the chest is known as the
   a. Bohr effect.
   b. bucket-handle effect.
   c. accessory effect.
   d. pump-handle effect

4. Which of the following muscles are used during inspiration?
   i. Diaphragm
   ii. External intercostal
   iii. Anterior serratus
   iv. External obliques
   v. Pectoralis major

   a. i, ii, iii
   b. ii, iii, iv
   c. iii, iv, v
   d. i, ii, iii, v
   e. All of the above

5. The points of origin for attachment of the diaphragm are
   i. sternal.
   ii. spinal.
   iii. costal.
   iv. phrenic.
   v. lumbar.

   a. i, ii, iii
   b. ii, iii, iv
   c. i, iii, v
   d. i, ii, iii, iv
   e. All of the above

6. The strength of a muscle is primarily determined by its
   a. power.
   b. endurance.
   c. size.
   d. innervation.
   e. environment.

7. The respiratory quotient for fat is
   a. 0.7.
   b. 0.8.
   c. 0.9.
   d. 1.0.
   e. 0.8–1.0.

2

▼

VENTILATION: AN OVERVIEW

1. NORMAL BREATHING
2. THE WORK OF BREATHING AND
   ITS EFFICIENCY
   Measuring the Work of Breathing

   Increases in the Work of
   Breathing
   Reducing the Work of Breathing
3. CONCLUSION

OBJECTIVES

1. Discuss the efficiency of breathing.

2. Distinguish the pressure volume curve from the pressure-volume loop.

3. List the common abnormalities in breathing function.

This chapter provides a brief overview of spontaneous ventilation, or breathing, the process by which oxygen is extracted from the environment and exchanged for expired carbon dioxide. The focus is on normal, healthy spontaneous ventilation, but instances in which this process is disrupted by stress and disease are also discussed, as is the need for mechanical ventilation.

▼ NORMAL BREATHING

Depending on body type and size, the volume of gas inspired and expired with each breath is approximately 400–600 mL and is known as a tidal volume (V_T). The consecutive breaths characteristic of spontaneous ventilation is known as **tidal breathing**. The number of breaths per minute also varies from one individual to another, normally varying between 12 and 18 breaths (**respiratory rate**, RR). The number of breaths per minute multiplied by the tidal vol-

Matthews LR: CARDIOPULMONARY ANATOMY AND PHYSIOLOGY. © 1996 Lippincott–Raven Publishers.

ume is known as the **minute volume**. These interrelated measures—tidal volume, tidal breathing, respiratory rate, and minute volume—can be assessed to determine the nature and relative efficiency of breathing.

Spontaneous ventilation could not occur without the successful interplay between the pressure, volume, and flow of the gases to be exchanged (see Figure 2-1 to see how those measures are captured on a flowmeter readout). Keep in mind that a volume of gas flows across a pressure gradient from areas of high pressure to areas of lower pressure. It is the continuously alternating shifts in pressure gradients between the interior of the lungs and the outside environment that both prompt and allow spontaneous ventilation to continue. Also, note that pleural pressures (which are described in more detail in Chapter 4) along with alveolar pressure reflect the intrathoracic changes that contribute to the work of ventilation.

Boyle's law (see Appendix 2) states that there is an inverse relationship between volume and pressure. In other words, when volume increases, pressure decreases. Figure 2-1a shows a decrease in intrathoracic pressure relative to atmospheric, or ambient, pressure. This results in a flow of gas entering the chest (inspiration). Exhaling the gas requires that the thoracic volume decrease. Remember, Boyle's law also states that when volume decreases, pressure increases. (The downward deflection indicates outgoing flow, measured in liters per second, whereas the upward deflection represents incoming flow.)

Figure 2-1b shows an increase in intrathoracic pressure relative to atmospheric pressure. This results in a flow of gas exiting the chest (expiration). (As volume increases, the line moves upward; it moves back down toward the zero point, or baseline, when the pressure decreases.)

Normally, exhalation is achieved by relaxation, during which the lung returns to its natural resting position due to its elastic recoil. However, mild abdominal contractions have been recorded even during quiet breathing. During stress, such as that accompanying physical exertion, expiratory muscles are recruited to shorten expiratory time by forcing expiration. This increases the rate at which the lung takes in oxygen and expels carbon dioxide; in short, it increases the respiratory rate. Normally, expiratory time (E) is two to three times longer than inspiratory time (I), giving an I:E ratio of 1:2–1:3. When respiratory rate is dramatically increased, the expiratory rate is shortened so that the resultant I:E ratio is closer to 1:1.

Figure 2-1c shows the pleural pressure changes seen during inspiration and expiration. Normal pleural pressure, which is measured midlung with the patient in an upright position, registers at approximately -5 cm H_2O. When inspiration proceeds, the chest wall moves outward and the diaphragm moves downward, pulling out on the lung and creating a greater negative pleural pressure (-8 to -9 cm H_2O). Then, as the chest relaxes and the diaphragm moves upward, the pressure returns to its baseline of -5 cm H_2O (average).

Figure 2-1d shows the changing alveolar pressure generated as the chest wall is pumped. Alveolar pressure moves above and below atmospheric pressure (1,032 cm H_2O at sea level) and is used as a zero baseline. The inspiratory pressure is negative, resulting in air movement into the lungs. The expiratory

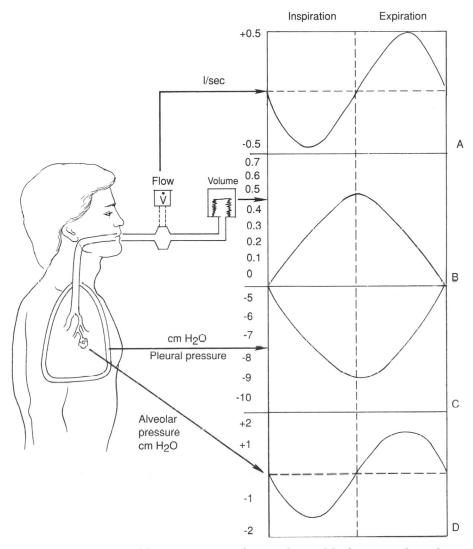

Figure 2-1.   Four possible monitor waveforms obtainable from one breathing cycle. (a) The flow waveform found during inspiration and expiration. Negative flow is recorded as gas flows into the lungs and positive flow is recorded as gas flows out of the lungs. (b) The volume waveform obtained as volume enters the lung and then is pushed back out. (c) The pressure waveform obtained when pleural pressure is monitored during inspiration and expiration. Note the greater negative pressure during inspiration. (d) The pressure waveform obtained while measuring alveolar pressure during inspriation and expiration. Notice the negative pressure resulting in gas entering the lungs and positive pressure resulting in gas exiting the lungs.

pressure is positive, resulting in gas movement out of the lung (chest). This changing alveolar pressure is the direct result of the inward and outward movement of the chest wall. The actual pressure needed to pull the lung outward is reflected only in pleural pressure and does not take into account any problems associated with chest wall stiffness (see Chapter 3).

▼ THE WORK OF BREATHING AND ITS EFFICIENCY

Work is required to move gas into and out of the lungs. For inspiration, this work is accomplished entirely by the muscles of ventilation. In normal, healthy subjects this movement of gas requires less than 5% of the total amount of oxygen used by the body for basal metabolic function. As you will recall from Chapter 1, this oxygen is chiefly consumed by the diaphragm and the external intercostals to power inspiration. The stored energy in the form of elastic recoil is used for expiration.

Work of breathing (the work required to take a single breath) is defined as the change in pleural pressure (ΔP) multiplied by the change in volume (ΔV):

$$\text{Work of breathing} = \Delta P \times \Delta V$$

The efficiency of breathing describes the metabolic cost for a given work output to effect a given gas exchange in the lung. When the actual quantity of gas being exchanged does not increase to keep pace with energy needs, efficiency begins to decline.

$$\text{Efficiency of breathing} = \text{total gas exchange } (O_2 \text{ uptake})/\text{gas consumed in the}$$

$$\text{act (cost of breathing)}$$

The work of breathing may increase or decrease in response to various physiological or pathophysiological changes. A decline in the efficiency of breathing is one of the hallmarks of pulmonary disease. When the oxygen consumption required for breathing becomes too great, mechanical ventilation may be prescribed to take over a portion of the work involved, or it may take over the work of breathing entirely. Mechanical ventilation effectively reduces the body's overall oxygen consumption. This buys valuable time needed to treat the underlying disease process.

Whether mechanical ventilation is prescribed, continued, or discontinued depends on how accurately the measurement of the work of breathing is performed.

Measuring the Work of Breathing

Figure 2-2 illustrates the changes in pleural pressure seen during inspiration and expiration, which result in a volume of gas entering and leaving the lung. When alveolar pressure is negative, volume will enter the lungs, and when alveolar pressure is positive, volume will exit the lungs.

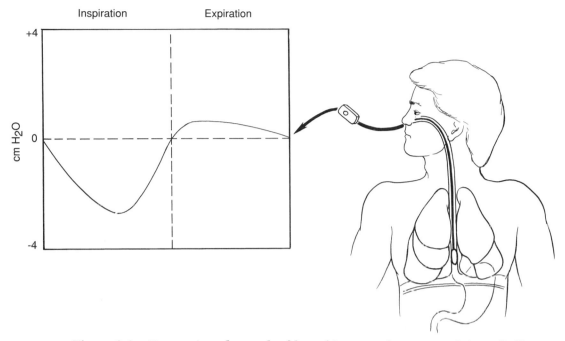

Figure 2-2. **To monitor the work of breathing, a catheter containing a balloon close to its tip is placed in the esophagus. Pressure is continuously monitored, providing a direct reflection of pleural pressure changes. Direct pleural pressure monitoring is almost impossible to accomplish.**

Because alveolar pressure reflects only the end result and not the work necessary to develop these pressures, pleural pressure must somehow be approximated. Because the esophagus passes directly into the chest cavity and sits in the mediastinum, pleural pressure can be approximated by monitoring esophageal pressure. When pressures needed for lung expansion change, the entire thoracic cavity is affected. Therefore, a pressure measurement inside the esophagus reflects the pressure required for breathing.

When the resistance to expansion of the lung is increased, the difference between alveolar pressure and pleural pressure (**transpulmonary pressure**) can be greatly increased:

$$\text{Transpulmonary pressure} = P_{alveolar} - P_{pleural}$$

This is because of the increased need for an outward pull on the lung as its *compliance* (ability to accommodate lung expansion) is reduced (see Chapter 3 for a more detailed discussion of compliance and resistance, two important forces that must be overcome for ventilation to occur).

Figure 2-3 is a graphic representation of combining pressure (x axis) and volume (y axis). The greater the area inside this pressure-volume curve, the greater the work the patient must do to breathe. Ongoing monitoring of this

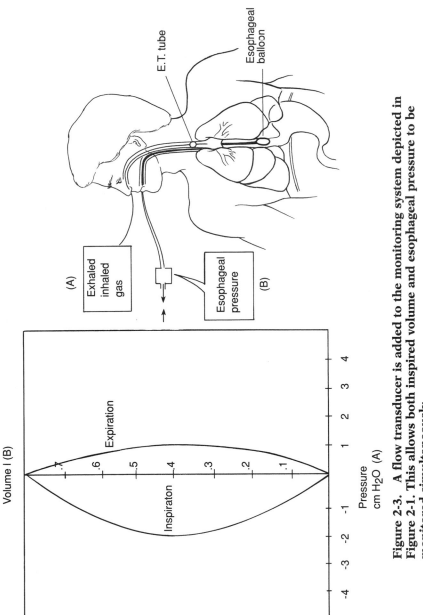

Figure 2-3. A flow transducer is added to the monitoring system depicted in Figure 2-1. This allows both inspired volume and esophageal pressure to be monitored simultaneously.

curve can give an excellent reflection of the patient's changing demands and the effectiveness of the therapy being provided. Stiff lungs and/or narrowing airways are reflected in a greater area inside the curve.

Increases in the Work of Breathing

During stress or disease, the ventilation reserve can be exhausted, and the oxygen made available by further increases in ventilation is entirely consumed by the ventilatory muscles. This makes any further increased effort wasted. If the increased work is caused by internal factors, it is referred to as *intrinsic*. If an external apparatus such as a mechanical ventilator is attached, additional work (*extrinsic*) may be required.

Pulmonary disease often results in a greater pressure needed to effect a given volume exchange. This results in more work or oxygen consumption needed to ventilate the lungs.

Reducing the Work of Breathing

In a healthy, exercising individual, the muscles of ventilation consume more oxygen and produce more carbon dioxide than they do when they are at rest. (At rest, the oxygen consumption of the muscles of ventilation is less than 10 mL/minute.) During exercise, there is a corresponding increase in oxygen uptake and carbon dioxide removal. This system keeps the cost of breathing down to less than 5% of the body's oxygen intake, even with major increases in ventilation.

Oxygen consumption can be greatly increased in disease, without a corresponding increase in ventilation for gas exchange. Energy is used up by trying to breathe through narrowing airways or stiff or tight lungs, common problems in respiratory diseases. This may result in an oxygen consumption equaling or exceeding 30% of the total oxygen uptake of the body. When this happens, there may not be enough oxygen remaining to sustain life, let alone fight off a disease process. When muscle work is dramatically increased because of narrowing airways or stiff lungs, drug administration is aimed at improving both problems. When muscle function is adversely affected, drug administration may be aimed at improving muscle function. When these approaches are ineffective in reducing the work required to breathe or in improving muscle function, the patient's life may be in jeopardy. In such cases, some form of mechanical support for breathing may be needed.

The overall goal of mechanical support in breathing must always be considered when evaluating how much help a patient needs. If the goal is to reverse ventilatory muscle fatigue, then near total rest is indicated, and completely removing the patient's load to breathe may be indicated. When muscle atrophy prevention is desired, then modest or partial removal of the patient work load may be indicated. If you wish to build up the patient's muscle strength, then short periods of high stress may prove effective. When building respiratory muscle endurance, protracted moderate work loads may be more effective in gradually reducing support until the patient regains complete control and does all of the work for himself or herself. Modern day ventilators are used to accomplish all of the above tasks with varying degrees of effectiveness.

The application of mechanical ventilatory support can reduce the muscle work required to breathe and assist the patient in reducing oxygen demand. The patient is then better able to fight off any existing disease process.

▼ CONCLUSION

Pressure, volume, and flow were all used to describe the changes observed during inspiration and expiration. The ways in which thoracic volume changes were explored allowed the reader to develop a clear understanding of the various mechanisms that are functioning during the breathing process.

This chapter also described the work required in the normal breathing process, as well as the factors associated with increased work of breathing and the methods of reducing it. The work of breathing is of concern to clinicians because it is directly related to disease and its progress. Now the reader should be able to forge ahead with confidence to study the therapeutic measures used to promote spontaneous ventilation. It is hoped that Chapter 2 has provided the reader with a solid foundation that will allow him or her to better appreciate how and why these therapeutic measures work.

The concepts of compliance and ventilation that were introduced in this chapter will be the focus of Chapter 3. These two factors are always at play in normal spontaneous ventilation. In fact, breathing can be characterized as a triumph over these factors. Abnormalities in compliance and fluctuations in resistance are also highly implicated in pulmonary disease. Whether these abnormalities are overcome may depend on the respiratory therapist's ability to identify them and correct them with the proper therapy.

❖ Review Questions

1. Which of the following laws describes the relationship between pressure and volume?
   a. Charles's
   b. Graham's
   c. Boyle's
   d. Gay-Lussac's
   e. Henry's
2. Expiratory time is normally _____ times longer than inspiratory time.
   a. 1–2
   b. 2–3
   c. 3–4
   d. 5–6
   e. 6–8

3. The oxygen demands for breathing are normally ____% of the total
    amount of oxygen consumed by the body.
    a. 1
    b. 5
    c. 10
    d. 20
    e. 30

3

CONTROL OF VENTILATION AND VENTILATORY PATTERN

Matthews LR: CARDIOPULMONARY ANATOMY AND PHYSIOLOGY. © 1996 Lippincott–Raven Publishers.

OBJECTIVES

1. Explain compliance and resistance and how they are implicated in spontaneous ventilation.

2. Characterize the relationship between tidal volume, respiratory rate, airway resistance, and pulmonary compliance.

3. Account for the variation in a pressure volume curve that occurs when airway resistance and pulmonary compliance are changed.

4. Define hysteresis.

5. Specify the roles played by $PaCO_2$, PaO_2, and pH in the chemical control of breathing.

6. Contrast and compare central and peripheral chemoreceptors.

7. Discuss the changes in PaO_2 and $PaCO_2$ that occur with the progressive development of lung disease.

8. Relate the neuronal control of breathing to both the dorsal and ventral respiratory groups.

9. Describe pneumotaxic regulation.

10. Illustrate the Hering-Breuer inflation reflex.

11. Characterize the apneustic center.

12. Describe the pulmonary receptors.

13. List and describe the abnormal breathing patterns.

As you will recall from the discussion of the work of breathing, the more pressure exerted to move a volume of gas, the more work involved. However, the work of breathing is designed to be performed with maximum efficiency under a variety of circumstances.

Spontaneous ventilation in healthy adults is deemed efficient if the entire process consumes no more than 5% of the oxygen (O_2) taken in by the lungs. The depth of breathing (**tidal volume**), the number of breaths per minute (**respiratory rate**), and the rhythm of the breathing pattern are all carefully regulated by physiological processes that are designed to keep the body's O_2 requirements to this 5% minimum, even under the most adverse conditions. It is when this standard cannot be met that abnormalities of ventilation are said to exist.

This chapter describes the three primary factors that can be manipulated to minimize the body's O_2 requirements:

1. The relationship between respiratory rate and tidal volume (airway resistance and lung compliance).
2. The necessary minute volume needed to ensure carbon dioxide (CO_2) removal and O_2 consumption.
3. The neuronal control of breathing, which assures a smooth, efficient pattern, or rhythm.

This chapter also presents a comprehensive description of the abnormal breathing patterns that can result from the various disease processes and traumas that can interrupt the normal physiological dynamics of breathing.

Our exploration of these topics begins with an examination of the relationship between two of the most important concepts related to spontaneous ventilation: compliance and resistance. The term **compliance** refers to the ease or difficulty with which the chest walls and lungs are moved to accommodate the inspiration or expiration of the gases exchanged in spontaneous ventilation. **Resistance**, on the other hand, describes the difficulty encountered while moving a flow of gas through airways that are narrow or constricted. Both of these factors must be overcome if normal breathing is to take place. Although we define these terms separately to identify specific underlying problems, they both contribute to the work of breathing.

▼ COMPLIANCE AND RESISTANCE

Compliance

Generally, we equate the compliance of a given body or organ with its distensibility, or stretchability. This quality is not to be confused with the related concept of *stiffness*, or *elasticity*, terms used interchangeably to describe the ability or tendency of a material to regain its shape after being stretched.

The term *compliance* is used to describe (1) an increase or decrease in elasticity and (2) the work required to expand the chest (chest wall, or thoracic, compliance) or lung (pulmonary compliance). Compliance is inversely related to pressure and work (i.e., as the pressure required to expand the chest increases, the compliance decreases).

$$\text{Compliance} = \frac{\text{Volume (L)}}{\text{Pressure (cm } H_2O)}$$

This volume is always expressed in liters per centimeter H_2O pressure and normally ranges between 0.1 and 0.2.

Example #1

$$\text{Tidal} = \text{volume 600 mL}$$
$$\text{Pressure required} = 3 \text{ cm } H_2O$$
$$\text{Compliance}^* = 600 \text{ mL/3 cm } H_2O$$
$$= 200 \text{ mL/cm } H_2O \text{ (or 0.2 L/cm } H_2O)$$

Example #2

$$Tidal\ volume = 600\ mL$$
$$Pressure\ required = 6\ cm\ H_2O$$
$$Compliance^* = 600\ mL/6\ cm\ H_2O$$
$$= 100\ mL/cm\ H_2O\ (or\ 0.1/cm\ H_2O)$$

In Example 1, the pulmonary compliance is twice as great as that in Example 2. It can be seen that the pressure in Example 2 is twice that in Example 1. This shows the inverse relationship between the pressure required to achieve a given volume and compliance (mL/cm H_2O). If the rib cage and/or surrounding tissues become less compliant (or more restrictive), more work is required for breathing.

Spontaneous Breathing

Although the lungs alone are almost twice as compliant as the lungs and chest wall combined, the work of breathing is a function of joint pulmonary and chest wall compliance.

Pulmonary compliance is associated with changes in intrapleural pressure. Generally a stiff, or noncompliant, lung results in greater negative intrapleural pressure, whereas a floppy, or very compliant, lung results in less negative pleural pressure. Because pleural pressure changes are reflective of lung compliance alone, there is generally no need to assess thoracic compliance separately although it must be taken into consideration. In any event, most of the disease processes affecting the pulmonary system have an impact on lung compliance and not thoracic wall compliance.

During a normal breath the rib cage is pulled up and out, and the diaphragm contracts to pull downward on the lungs. If it is more difficult to pull the lungs outward, then a greater negative pressure will develop in the pleural space (potential space) (Figure 3-1). Remember that during spontaneous breathing, measurements reflecting pleural pressures (e.g., esophageal pressure) are indicative of the work required to expand the lung only, not the thorax (Figure 3-1). Work can be increased as a result of decreasing chest wall compliance, but chest wall compliance can be much more difficult to assess.

Factors Causing Abnormalities in Compliance

The normal compliance of the lungs can be affected by the presence of any number of disease processes or conditions. Among the conditions that lead to increased compliance are those that cause destruction of lung tissue such as emphysema. Conditions that lead to decreased compliance include those that are responsible for long-term irritation and inflammation, such as fibrosis or tissue scarring, and those that impede lung expansion, such as kyphosis, which decreases compliance because it restricts chest wall movement.

---

*Compliance is commonly expressed in liters per centimeter H_2O; to convert the values provided to liters, simply divide by 1,000.

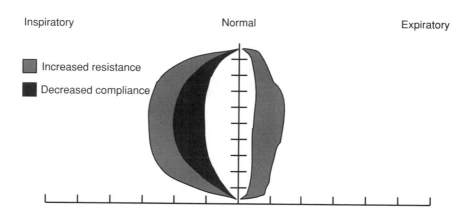

Figure 3-1.   Pressure volume curve. As the lungs become stiff (less compliant), more pressure is required to pull them outward. An esophageal balloon can be placed inside the esophagus within the mediastinum. This pressure monitor reflects pleural pressure to indicate the pressure required for breathing (see Chapter 1).

Resistance

Changes in intrathoracic volume result in pressure changes with a corresponding flow of gas. Gas always moves across a pressure gradient from high to low pressure. Thus, it follows that negative pressure in the chest prompts a flow of gas into the lung, whereas positive pressure inside the chest results in a flow of gas out of the lung.

$$\dot{V} = \frac{P_1 - P_2}{R}$$

where $\dot{V}$ = gas flow
R = airway resistance
P_1 = pressure initially
P_2 = pressure downstream

Keep in mind that work is required to move a volume of gas through the airways. This work is reflected in the pressure required to move that flow of gas through a particular passageway. As the pressure increases, the work also increases, making it harder to breathe.

The ease or difficulty of breathing is affected at least in part by the airway's natural resistance to the flow of gases, which is expressed as follows:

Example #3

(pressure) (flow)
Airway resistance = 1.0 cm H_2O/L/sec
(R_{AW})

This means that 1.0 cm H_2O pressure is required to move a flow of gas at a rate of 1 L/sec. The same amount of pressure is required to move this flow of gas either into or out of the lung. If the gas flow is increased to 2 L/sec, it would take 2.0 cm H_2O pressure to move (ignoring the possible development of turbulent flow explained in Chapter 4).

R_{AW} = Pressure required (cm H_2O)/Gas flow (L/sec)
= 2 cm H_2O/2 L/sec
= 1 cm H_2O/L/sec

Under normal circumstances we can measure both the pressure due to resistance (sometimes referred to as back pressure), as well as inspiratory flow. The combination of these two values gives us a resistance in centimeters H_2O per liter per second. Therefore, if the pressure due to resistance is measured at 2 cm H_2O and the inspiratory flow is measured at 0.5 L/sec, the airway resistance would be calculated as follows:

Example #4

R_{AW} = Pressure due to gas flow resistance/Inspiratory flow
= 2 cm H_2O/0.5 L/sec
= 4 cm H_2O/L/sec

How resistance affects flow through the airways is calculated as follows:

$$\dot{V}_I = [P_M - P_A]/R_{AW}$$

where $\dot{V}_I$ is inspiratory flow, P_M is the mouth pressure, P_A is the alveolar pressure, and R_{AW} is the airway resistance.

Figure 3-2 demonstrates the impact that resistance has on flow. When resistance is doubled, flow is effectively cut in half.

Example #5 (see Figure 3-2a)

P_M = 0 cm H_2O (ambient or atmospheric)
P_A = -3 cm H_2O (negative pressure generated by the increased thoracic volume during inspiration)
R_{AW} = 2 cm H_2O/L/sec (back pressure generated by the flow passing through the airway)
$\dot{V}_I$ = [0 $-$ (-3) cm H_2O]/2 cm H_2O/L/sec
= 3/2 L/sec
= 1.5 L/sec, the flow that would be generated given the pressure difference across the airway and the airway resistance.

During expiration, flow must reverse direction to exit the airway. Thus, the relationships outlined above will change in the following manner:

$$\dot{V}_E = [P_A - P_M]/R_{AW}$$

where $\dot{V}_E$ is expiratory flow.

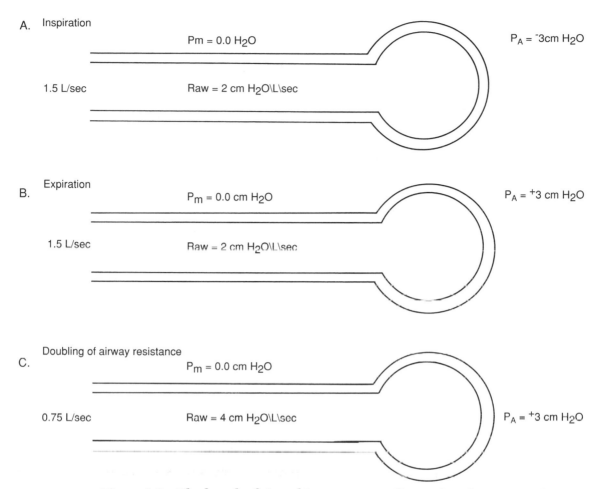

A. Inspiration

Pm = 0.0 H₂O $P_A = ^-3cm\ H_2O$

1.5 L/sec   Raw = 2 cm H₂O\L\sec

B. Expiration

$P_m = 0.0\ cm\ H_2O$ $P_A = ^+3\ cm\ H_2O$

1.5 L/sec   Raw = 2 cm H₂O\L\sec

C. Doubling of airway resistance

$P_m = 0.0\ cm\ H_2O$

0.75 L/sec   Raw = 4 cm H₂O\L\sec $P_A = ^+3\ cm\ H_2O$

Figure 3-2. **The length of time this pressure gradient exists determines the size of the tidal volume: (a) inspiration; (b) expiration; (c) impact of resistance on flow (when resistance is doubled, flow is effectively cut in half).**

Example #6 (see Figure 3-2b)

$$P_A = +3\ cm\ H_2O$$
$$P_M = 0\ cm\ H_2O$$
$$R_{AW} = 2\ cm\ H_2O/L/sec$$
$$\dot{V}_E = [+3\ cm\ H_2O - 0\ cm\ H_2O]/2\ cm\ H_2O/L/sec$$
$$= [3\ cm\ H_2O]/2\ cm\ H_2O/L/sec$$
$$= 3/2\ L/sec$$
$$= 1.5\ L/sec$$

If airway resistance increases as a result of reduced airway caliber (diameter), the amount of pressure or work required to move a flow of gas through that airway will be increased accordingly.

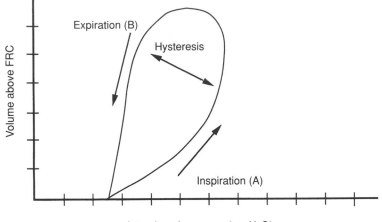

Figure 3-3.   This curve graphically depicts the work required to breathe as the combined result of compliance and resistance. The functional residual capacity (FRC) denotes the gas remaining in the lungs at the end of a passive exhalation. Hysteresis is the term used to describe the difference in the inspiratory and expiratory curves.

Figure 3-3 indicates that the expiratory flow curve (B) requires less pressure to achieve than the inspiratory curve (A). The difference in these two pressures is known as hysteresis. Mathematically, the same amount of pressure is required to move a volume of gas, whether the movement is into or out of the lungs. However, the work required to inflate the chest for inspiration must be generated entirely by the muscles of inspiration. The force required to expire a volume of gas is primarily generated by the elastic recoil of the lungs and relaxation of the diaphragm with displacement of the abdominal contents; in healthy individuals, this requires little, if any, work.

As described in Chapter 2, the work required to breathe can be monitored in patients experiencing ventilatory failure. *Ambient,* or *baseline,* pressure is used as a center point against which the pressure required to move a given volume of gas into the chest is compared. The y axis in Figure 3-4a shows the tidal volume developed, and the x axis shows the required negative and positive pressures needed to inhale and exhale. The area within the curve changes to reflect any changes in airway resistance or lung compliance. Figure 3-4a–c shows the changes that may be encountered in clinical practice.

▼ RELATIONSHIPS BETWEEN RESPIRATORY RATE AND TIDAL VOLUME

Each time the muscles of inspiration contract, work is accomplished. More work, and thus more energy and O_2, is required when the target tidal volume is large (Figure 3-5). When compliance of the thorax is less than the normal

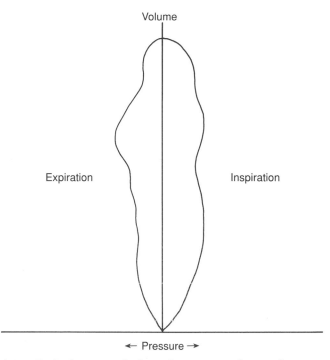

Volume

Expiration   Inspiration

A   ← Pressure →

Figure 3-4. **(a) A relatively normal pleural pressure change from expiration to inspiration. (b) This graph, which represents low lung compliance with a high negative pressure required to inspire and an expiratory resistance, is indicative of an increase in the work of breathing. (c) This graphic depiction is also indicative of labor-intensive spontaneous ventilation. It represents the normal negative pressure required to inspire and a high expiratory resistance with a high pressure required to exhale.**

range of 0.1–0.2 L/cm H_2O, greater pressure is needed to develop a tidal volume of the same size. The body naturally responds to this decrease in thoracic compliance by reducing the size of the tidal volume, thus cutting down on the amount of O_2 and energy needed to breathe.

When the tidal volume is reduced, alveolar ventilation for a given breath is reduced, which requires a compensatory increase in minute volume. Although a smaller tidal volume uses less energy than a large one, this energy savings is countered to some degree by the need to take more breaths than usual to keep up with the required gas exchange. Small tidal volumes also result in the need to breathe faster, which increases the inspiratory flow of gas.

During inspiration and expiration, gas must flow through the airways that lead to the lungs. Work is required to overcome the friction encountered when air rubs up against the walls of these airways. The caliber of a normal, healthy airway opening is large enough to accommodate with ease the flow of gas with a minimal expenditure of energy. When the airway is small, more gas

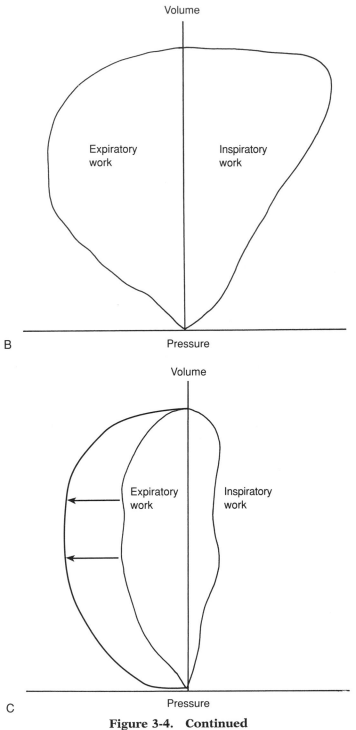

Figure 3-4. Continued

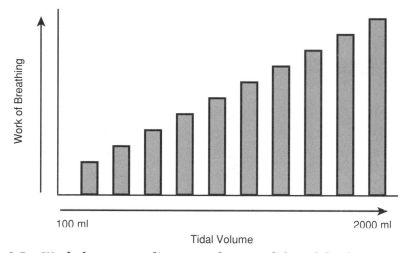

Figure 3-5.   Work due to compliance. As the size of the tidal volume increases, the work, or energy expenditure, increases.

comes in contact with its walls, thus increasing the work needed to move gas through the tube.

The caliber of the airways is to some extent under the control of the smooth muscles that line their interiors. These muscles are capable of relaxing (*bronchodilation*) or constricting (*bronchoconstriction*). Also, mucus produced through stimulation or irritation of the airways can affect the caliber of the airways by inducing bronchoconstriction. Respiratory therapy is often directed at reducing the resultant inflammation by eliminating the secretions or removing the underlying cause of irritation. Bronchodilators also may be given to relax the smooth muscle and increase the internal diameter of the airways.

Airway resistance, which is normally 1–2 cm H_2O/L/sec, is a determinant of the amount of work required for spontaneous ventilation. The smaller the airway, the greater the pressure requirement to move a volume of gas per unit of time. Imagine the work it would require to breathe through a small straw versus that needed to breathe through a large garden hose. Breathing through the straw, which offers greater airway resistance, would be appreciably more difficult. In order to meet the incessant demands of spontaneous ventilation, the body somehow has to minimize the work needed to move a flow of gas through airways of all sizes.

As the rate at which we inspire increases or the airway gets smaller, the work required (measured in terms of O_2 consumed) increases. (See Figure 3-6 for a graphic representation of how the work of breathing grows with the increase in inspiratory flow.) At first glance, it seems to make sense that inhaling slowly would reduce the work of breathing. But a slow inspiratory flow reduces the overall exhalation time. This effect demands that we take in a larger

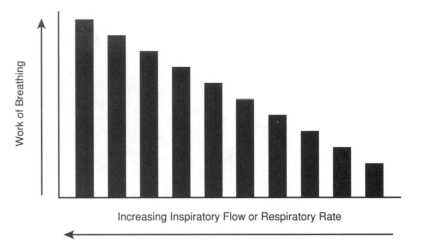

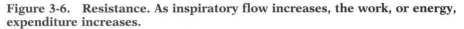

Figure 3-6.   Resistance. As inspiratory flow increases, the work, or energy, expenditure increases.

tidal volume, which in turn leads to greater exertion as the chest is pushed out farther.

Figure 3-6 shows that the rate of inspiratory flow and the size of tidal volume are inversely related to one another. In other words, small tidal volumes require higher respiratory rates and inspiratory flow, whereas low inspiratory flow requires larger tidal volumes. In order to maintain the natural efficiency of spontaneous ventilation, an optimum balance must be achieved between respiratory rate and tidal volume.

If the airway caliber is reduced, more work is required to move a flow of gas through the airway. Therefore, a slower flow with a larger tidal volume minimizes the work of breathing (Figure 3-7).

If the chest were to become less compliant, it would take more energy to inspire a given size tidal volume. In this case, a smaller tidal volume and a higher respiratory rate minimizes the work of breathing. Diseases that affect the caliber of the airway (e.g., asthma or bronchitis) or increase the stiffness of the chest (e.g., pulmonary fibrosis) change the relationship between tidal volume and respiratory rate (Table 3-1).

To summarize, the muscles of breathing "normally" perform work to support inspiration, not expiration. This work can be divided into three categories, two of which have already been discussed:

1. The work required to expand the lungs (compliance).
2. The work required to move gas through the airways (resistance).
3. The tissue-resistive work, or the work required to overcome the viscosity of the lung and chest wall parenchyma (interstitium of the lung). Normally, this work is negligible in comparison with the expenditure of energy required in the first two circumstances.

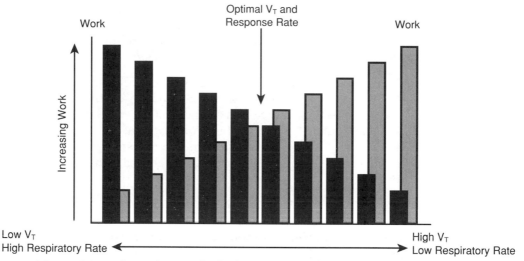

Figure 3-7. The point at which the work of breathing is minimized is represented as the balance between inspiratory flow and tidal volume size.

TABLE 3-1 Physiological Response		
	Tidal Volume	Respiratory Rate
Emphysema compliance ↑	↑	↓
Kyphoscoliosis compliance ↓	↓	↑
Asthma resistance ↑	↑	↓
Bronchodilator therapy resistance ↓	↓	↑

(It is held to <5% of the total energy expenditure of the body, even during the maximum exertion of exercise.)

In any case, the relationship between tidal volume and respiratory rate gravitates toward the point where a minimum energy expenditure is required. A change in the size of a patient's tidal volume and/or rate of breathing are early indications of respiratory abnormalities.

In the end stages of respiratory disease, the work of breathing can decrease dramatically. In some acute and chronic diseases, the work can become incompatible with life, and mechanical ventilation may be necessary (described in Chapter 1).

▼ THE CHEMICAL CONTROL OF BREATHING

The goal of ventilation, whether spontaneous or mechanical, is to acquire adequate quantities of O_2, remove sufficient quantities of CO_2, and maintain the appropriate hydrogen ion ($[H^+]$) concentration in body fluids (see Chapter 12). It is for these reasons that the respiratory centers for ventilation are so responsive to O_2, CO_2, and extracellular pH. The following physiological responses are present under normal circumstances:

1. Increase in $[H^+]$ concentration causes an increase in ventilation.
2. Increase in CO_2 levels causes an increase in ventilation.
3. Decrease in O_2 levels causes an increase in ventilation, provided it occurs outside the central nervous system.
4. Decreased O_2 levels in the central nervous system result in depression of the respiratory centers and therefore a decrease in ventilation.

There are areas in the brain and in the major arteries that are sensitive to CO_2, O_2, and $[H^+]$ concentration. These regions, known as chemoreceptors, are divided into two primary groups: the central and the peripheral. They are so designated for their residence either within or peripheral to the central nervous system.

Central Chemoreceptors

A chemoreceptor area is located in the *medulla*, the lower portion of the brainstem. This area is sensitive to changes in blood CO_2 and, to a lesser degree, blood $[H^+]$ concentration. It is responsible for stimulating other portions of the respiratory center to increase both the rate and depth of breathing (Figure 3-8). It is thought that the most important direct stimulant of this center is cerebrospinal fluid (CSF) $[H^+]$ concentration. There are two possible avenues for this stimulation:

1. $[H^+]$ in the blood has a considerably reduced effect on stimulation of the central chemoreceptors because blood H^+ ions are not readily soluble in lipid-based membranes such as the blood–brain barrier. Blood pH does have an impact on ventilation, but when we compare its effect to CO_2, its relative importance is diminished.
2. There is a direct relationship between CO_2, $[H^+]$ concentration, and an increased stimulus to breathe.

The stimulating effect of increasing arterial CO_2 ($PaCO_2$) level peaks in a few minutes and then gradually decreases over time. This gradual decrease over time is thought to be the result of bicarbonate buffering in the CSF. An acute response can be seen, followed by a weaker chronic response.

It is evident that $PaCO_2$ plays the main role in normal minute ventilation control. The normal arterial range is 35–45 mmHg (content is approximately 49 mL/dL). However, one must remember that this stimulation is indirect in that it changes the CSF $[H^+]$ concentration to stimulate the central chemoreceptors.

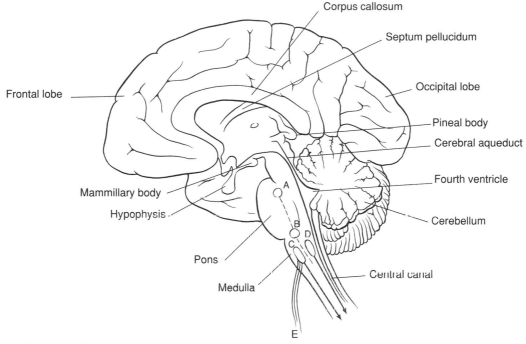

A   Pneumotaxic center
B   Apneustic center
C   Ventral respiratory group
D   Dorsal respiratory group
E   Vagus and glossopharyngeal nerves

Figure 3-8. CO_2 diffuses across the blood–brain barrier into the CSF. Once in the CSF, it combines with water to produce carbonic acid and reduce the fluid pH. It is the reduced pH of the CSF that directly stimulates the central chemoreceptors to cause increased ventilations and reduce $PaCO_2$. $PaCO_2 \rightarrow CO_2 + H_2O \leftrightarrow H_2CO_3 \leftrightarrow H^+ + HCO_3^-$; $[H^+]$ and pH (in the CSF); causes increased ventilation to bring $PaCO_2$ back to normal.

Peripheral Chemoreceptors

The peripheral chemoreceptors are sensory organs or nerve endings located outside the central nervous system (Figure 3-9) that are stimulated by and react to chemical stimuli. The *carotid* and *aortic bodies* are the chemoreceptors with which we will concern ourselves. Note that in normal, healthy subjects the peripheral chemoreceptors play little or no role in the control of ventilation. Peripheral chemoreceptors become significant only when O_2 levels in the blood decrease to a critical level.

The carotid bodies are located in the bifurcations of the common carotid arteries. The *afferent nerves*, which transmit impulses from the periphery to the central nervous system, pass through Hering's nerves to the *glossopharyngeal nerves* and then to the *dorsal respiratory group* of the medulla. The aortic

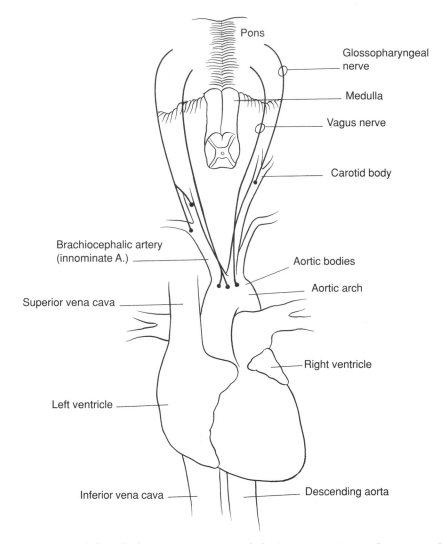

Figure 3-9.   Peripheral chemoreceptors and their connective pathways to the brain.

bodies are located along the aortic arch. The afferent nerves pass through the vagus into the dorsal respiratory group. These chemoreceptors are very vascular and receive a supply of blood from the adjacent artery which far exceeds the local cellular demand.

The partial pressure of O_2 (PaO_2) in arterial blood has no direct stimulatory effect on the central chemoreceptors. In fact, central hypoxia (decreased O_2 in inspired air) actually depresses ventilation. However, hypoxemia (inadequate oxygenation of blood) stimulates the peripheral chemoreceptors but not until the PaO_2 decreases to <50–60 mmHg. This is primarily because of the coinciding decrease in the O_2-carrying content of the blood (i.e., arterial O_2 content is not significantly reduced until the PaO_2 is $<50–60$ mmHg).

The blood supply of peripheral receptors is extremely high. As a result, relatively little O_2 is removed from this blood as it passes through the receptor. This allows blood in the receptors to have an O_2 content close to that of arterial blood, making the receptors responsive to arterial, not venous, O_2 levels (see Chapter 7). Serious **hypotension** (reduction in systolic and diastolic pressure) also can stimulate these receptors by decreasing blood supply and thus O_2 supply to the receptors. The exact mechanism of stimulation of this nerve center is unclear.

An increase in either $PaCO_2$ or $[H^+]$ concentration directly stimulates the peripheral chemoreceptors to increase ventilation. But the most significant impact of both of these factors is on the central receptors.

Inhibition of the Drive to Breathe

There are two significant factors that can inhibit the drive to breathe in disease states:

1. Decreased $PaCO_2$
2. Decreased $[H^+]$ concentration

If the $PaCO_2$ and $[H^+]$ concentration decrease at the same time, PaO_2 decreases. The result is a cancelling out of respiratory center stimulation, making the $PaCO_2$ mechanism insignificant.

However, if the $PaCO_2$ and $[H^+]$ concentration increase at the same time, the PaO_2 decreases. All three mechanisms result in a significant increase in the drive to breathe.

Chemoreceptor Role in Health and Disease

As was stated previously, the peripheral receptors play a negligible role in the control of ventilation. It is the combined effect of CO_2 and $[H^+]$ concentration on the central receptors that plays the primary role in spontaneous ventilation.

In chronic disease, such as emphysema and bronchitis, CO_2 levels may become chronically elevated and, in time, become less significant in their ability to stimulate breathing. O_2 may then become a major player in the mechanism that regulates ventilation. Under these circumstances, a decrease in arterial PaO_2 may cause a fivefold increase in ventilation.

Respiratory failure can develop quickly (as, for example, in a drug overdose) or over a period of years (as is the case with emphysema). The first indications of failure can be seen in a gradually decreasing PaO_2 (Figure 3-10). When the PaO_2 decreases to 50–60 mmHg, the peripheral chemoreceptors stimulate the drive centers to increase ventilation in the lungs. Once this begins to occur, $PaCO_2$ decreases (decreasing CSF $[H^+]$ concentration) and inhibits the drive to breathe. These two forces tend to cancel each other out.

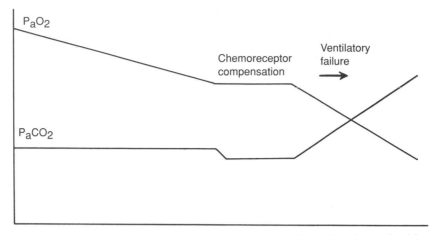

Figure 3-10.   Progressive changes are seen in O_2 and CO_2 levels in the blood as the respiratory system begins to fail.

The increased work of breathing that accompanies this increased drive is also somewhat self-defeating. The end result is a nominal decrease in $PaCO_2$ with a leveling out of the decreasing PaO_2. This may remain unchanged until the disease process progresses further. When compensation is no longer effective, the $PaCO_2$ will begin to climb and the PaO_2 will begin to decrease. Over time, the kidneys will begin to compensate for the increasing $PaCO_2$ and $[H^+]$ by retaining bicarbonate (HCO_3^-). This retained HCO_3^-, which reduces the drive to breathe, has a tendency to cancel out the effect of elevated CO_2, which increases the drive to breathe. When this occurs, the low O_2 levels are detected through the peripheral chemoreceptors and at that point become a significant stimulus in the drive to breathe. O_2 therapy administered to these patients reduces the stimulation to breathe and may actually have a detrimental effect. As in most situations, O_2 concentration should be kept as low as possible to maximize benefit and minimize side effects.

▼ NEURONAL CONTROL OF BREATHING

We have already described the relationship between the size of the tidal volume and the breathing rate required to provide a given volume of alveolar ventilation. The amount of O_2 required and the amount of CO_2 produced determine the minute volume.

In order to minimize the effort required to breathe, the body must set up a regulatory system that ensures a smooth, rhythmic breathing pattern. This smooth electrical control over the muscles of ventilation prevents sudden and erratic inspiration and expiration, which effectively keeps O_2 consumption to a minimum.

The rhythm of breathing is normally controlled by the respiratory centers, which are actually distinct groups of neurons located in the *pons* and *medulla oblongata* (Figure 3-8). Higher center control can override this function at any time because we have the ability to consciously vary our breathing pattern at will.

The respiratory center can be divided into three primary groups:

1. Dorsal respiratory group (primarily inspiration) located in the dorsal portion of the medulla oblongata (D in Figure 3-8).
2. Ventral respiratory group (inspiration and expiration) located in the ventrolateral part of the medulla oblongata (C in Figure 3-8).
3. Pneumotaxic center (rate and pattern) located dorsally in the superior aspects of the pons (A in Figure 3-8).

The Dorsal Respiratory Group

The vast majority of these neurons are located within the nucleus of the *tractus solitarius* of the medulla. This is an area of sensory termination for both the vagal nerve (this mixed nerve carries motor and sensory functions) and the *glossopharyngeal nerves* (pertaining to the tongue and pharynx). It imports information from the peripheral chemoreceptors. This region in the medulla is almost entirely responsible for stimulating the muscles of inspiration during quiet, normal breathing.

The electrical signal emitted from this region has a ramplike representation (Figure 3-11). This characteristic pattern of electrical activity results in a smooth, gradual increase in thoracic volume, which prevents inspiration from degenerating into an erratic series of gasps. The nervous signal transmitted from this region can control the following:

1. The rate of increase of the ramp, increasing the intrathoracic volume quickly, thereby making inspiration very quick when needed.
2. The point at which the signal stops and starts again, increasing or decreasing breathing rate.

The normal passivity of expiration is the result of the absence of stimulation from this area and is captured in the depressions between the rounded ramplike protrusions in Figure 3-11.

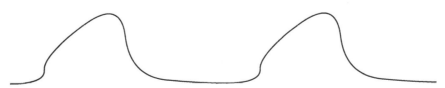

Figure 3-11.   The raised, ramplike "waves" indicate smooth, rhythmic inhalation. The "trough" between the inhalations represents the negligible work of expiration.

The Ventral Respiratory Group

This area of the medulla oblongata is important when breathing becomes more active (i.e., with the exertion brought on by disease or exercise). These neurons are present almost entirely within the *nucleus ambiguous* and the *nucleus retro-ambiguous*, which are associated with the glossopharyngeal and vagal nerves. These neurons are

1. almost totally inactive during passive breathing.
2. probably not involved in the rhythmic stimulation that provides a smooth breathing pattern.
3. active during labored breathing or exercise.
4. involved in both inspiration and expiration, depending on the region of the ventral respiratory group.
5. important in providing stimulus to the muscles of expiration for forced expiratory maneuvers.

The Pneumotaxic Center

The role of the pneumotaxic center appears to be one of inhibition. When signals leaving the pneumotaxic center are strong, inspiration is short; when the signal is weak, inspiration is longer. The result of this is a change in breathing rate. A strong signal from the pneumotaxic center results in an increased breathing rate, and a weak signal from the pneumotaxic center results in a decreased breathing rate.

The Hering-Breuer Inflation Reflex

These receptors are located in the wall of the bronchi and *bronchioles*. They are responsible for providing information to the respiratory center regarding the state of inflation of the lungs. They transmit signals through the vagus nerve (10th cranial nerve) into the dorsal respiratory group. When the lungs become overinflated, a signal is sent to the respiratory center to switch off inspiration. During quiet, normal breathing these receptors do not play a significant role. They may become a part of the control of breathing when tidal volume increases by three- or fourfold its normal rate.

The Apneustic Center

This center is located in the lower pons. It appears to be involved in turning off inspiration. Removal of its influence results in a long uninterrupted inspiration of near-maximum proportion (apneusis) with only occasional short expiratory gasps. The significance of this center during normal breathing is not known (Figure 3-12).

Pulmonary Receptors

The respiratory system contains a number of receptors that can provide afferent information to the respiratory centers:

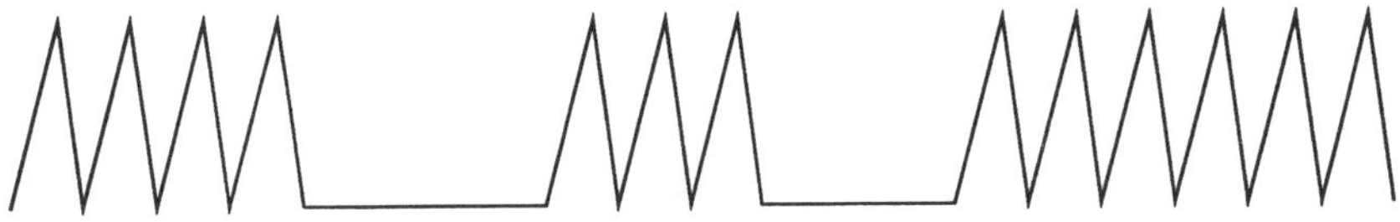

Figure 3-12. Apnea.

1. Stretch receptors
2. Irritant receptors
3. J receptors
4. Airway receptors
5. Joint and muscle receptors
6. Arterial baroreceptors
7. Pain receptors

Stretch Receptors

These receptors, which are located on the periphery of the lung, respond to pulmonary distention, or stretch. Stimulation of these receptors increases expiratory time and therefore decreases respiratory rate. This reflex was described earlier as the Hering-Breuer reflex.

Irritant Receptors

Located between the epithelial cells that line the airway, these receptors respond to the inhalation of noxious substances or severe environmental changes. The vagus nerve carries receptor impulses to the brain. The response is bronchospasm and hyperpnea (increased respiratory rate that is deeper than normal).

J Receptors

Known as juxtareceptors, these receptors are thought to exist in the alveolar walls. Pulmonary edema seems to stimulate these receptors to cause rapid, shallow breathing. They also may play a role in the sensation of shortness of breath (dyspnea). Impulses from these receptors reach the brain through the vagus nerve.

Airway Receptors

The nose, nasopharynx, larynx, and trachea have touch sensors. Stimulation of these receptors results in sneezing, coughing, bronchospasm, and laryngospasm. This is an attempt to inhibit the intrusion of foreign substances (see Chapter 15).

Joint and Muscle Receptors

Receptors found in the joints and muscles seem to play a role in the stimulation of ventilation, especially in the early stages of exercise. For example, the intercostal muscles and the diaphragm can sense muscle stretch and affect the strength of contraction in the following breath. These receptors also may play a role in the feeling of dyspnea.

Arterial Baroreceptors

Increased arterial blood pressure can result in hypoventilation, and decreased arterial blood pressure can cause hyperventilation. This reflex results through stimulation of the aortic and carotid sinus baroreceptors.

Pain

Pain can trigger apnea and subsequent hyperventilation. The mechanism by which this is achieved is poorly understood.

▼ BREATHING PATTERNS

Abnormal Breathing Patterns

The normal breathing pattern (eupnea) is generally smooth, regular, and subtle. A number of diseases or syndromes manifest themselves in part as abnormal breathing patterns. It is important for respiratory care professionals to recognize these abnormal patterns as indicative of disease processes. This section describes the following abnormal breathing patterns and their possible causes:

1. Cheyne-Stokes
2. Acute cerebral edema
3. Kussmaul's
4. Biots
5. Sleep apnea: central and obstructive
6. Apneustic
7. Paradoxic
8. Valsalva maneuver
9. Muller maneuver
10. Vagal
11. Coupled or grouped
12. Frog
13. Ataxic
14. Paradoxic reflex of head

Cheyne-Stokes

This breathing pattern is a combination of apnea and hyperventilation (Figure 3-13). This combination of hyper- and hypoventilation results from a delay in

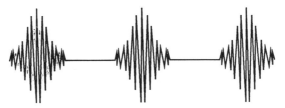

Figure 3-13.   Cheyne-Stokes breathing pattern, characterized by alternating hyperventilation and apnea.

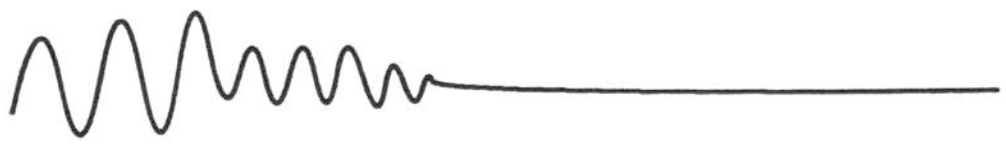

Figure 3-14.   Acute cerebral edema can disrupt normal ventilation and ultimately lead to apnea.

the blood traveling from the lungs to the brain, or brainstem damage resulting in a change in feedback sensitivity to CSF [H$^+$] concentration. The blood flow delay is most commonly related to cardiac failure. Hypoxia also may cause Cheyne-Stokes breathing by increasing central sensitivity to cause this irregular pattern.

Acute Cerebral Edema

If the brain is traumatized, the resulting swelling (edema) can compress the cerebral arteries to impede blood supply. This can inactivate or destroy neurons in the respiratory center, causing apnea (Figure 3-14). Mannitol can be used to remove fluid from the brain osmotically and to reduce swelling to improve blood supply.

Kussmaul's Breathing

This pattern of rapid, deep breathing is most commonly associated with a diabetic acidosis (Figure 3-15). It is the body's compensatory attempt to remove acid in the form of CO_2.

Biots Breathing

This is a breathing pattern with irregular periods of apnea interposed with runs of four to six deep breaths of identical size (Figure 3-16). It is often associated with increased intracranial pressure (which can be caused by any trauma that induces brain swelling) or midbrain lesions, tumors, or cerebral infarct.

Sleep Apnea: Central and Obstructive

Apnea is the cessation of breathing for a period of time that is characterized by ineffective inspiratory muscle effort (Figure 3-12). It can occur during sleep and is classified as either central or obstructive.

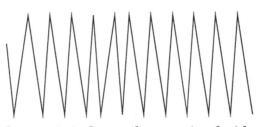

Figure 3-15.   The characteristic deep spikes associated with rapid, deep Kussmaul's breathing.

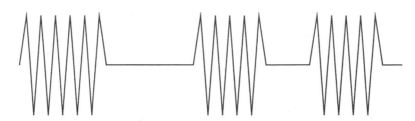

Figure 3-16.   Biots breathing is characterized by irregular periods of apnea interspersed with bouts of normal inhalations of groups of four to six deep breaths.

Central sleep apnea is the cessation of breathing resulting from the failure of the respiratory center. (This form of apnea is still poorly understood.) It can be a result of central nervous system abnormalities such as encephalitis, brainstem infarction, and bulbar poliomyelitis. Its idiopathic form is sometimes referred to as Ondine's curse. Current theories suggest that abnormalities in the control of breathing may place infants at particular risk of sudden infant death syndrome (SIDS).

Obstructive sleep apnea, which results from the closure or collapse of the pharynx, glottis, or larynx, is fairly well understood. This disorder is sometimes referred to as Pickwickian syndrome (after a Dickens character) and is commonly associated with obesity, collapsing of the throat, hypersomnolence, hypoxemia, and right heart failure. The possibility of a mixed disorder also exists if the individual exhibits both obstructive and central apnea.

Sleep apnea is particularly dangerous because it can go undetected for an extended period and thus result in death. The adult form (Ondine's curse) requires conscious control of ventilation to maintain $PaCO_2$ levels. SIDS is a fatal form of apnea that affects infants.

Apneustic Breathing
A patient engaged in this form of breathing exhibits sustained inspiratory effort, with irregular and brief expirations (Figure 3-17). This pattern is indicative of an imbalance in the neurons responsible for regulating rhythm.

Paradoxic Breathing
Paradoxic breathing results from a breach in the integrity of the chest wall or from the discoordination of the muscles of ventilation. The chest wall can move

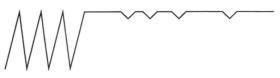

Figure 3-17.   The sustained inspiratory effort associated with apneustic breathing.

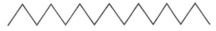

Figure 3-18.   Paradoxic breathing.

inward during inspiration and outward during exhalation. This motion can severely inhibit the ability to change intrathoracic pressure and create the necessary movement of gas in and out of the lungs during breathing, resulting in hypoventilation (Figure 3-18). This may result from a **flail chest** or intercostal diaphragmatic discoordination, also known as **respiratory alternans** (see Chapter 1).

The Valsalva Maneuver

This is more of a voluntary manipulation than a breathing pattern. This maneuver is achieved when contracted muscles of expiration create pressure against a closed glottis. This occurs during coughing, the instant before the glottis opens to expel unwanted contents, or during lifting.

The Muller Maneuver

Again, this is more of a maneuver than a breathing pattern. It results from contraction of the muscles of inspiration against a closed glottis.

Vagal Breathing

This slow, deep breathing pattern may come about when vagal afferents are interrupted.

Coupled or Grouped Breathing

This pattern is characterized by two or three breaths separated by periods of apnea of about 3–5 seconds' duration. The irregular blood gas levels experienced at high levels may prompt this ventilatory response (see Chapter 14).

Frog Breathing

Frog breathing, or glossopharyngeal ventilation, is effective when practiced by patients in whom the muscles of ventilation have been paralyzed but the muscles of swallowing (glossopharyngeal) have remained intact. Gulps of air are literally taken into the mouth and passed down into the lungs. This results in a steplike inflation of the lungs. Once an appropriate number of gulps has been taken, the patient passively exhales. This ventilatory technique is generally effective when coupled with very weak breathing or a cough.

Ataxic Breathing

This discoordinated breathing pattern, which results in irregular frequency and tidal volumes, may afflict infants during sleep or result from central nervous system lesions.

Paradoxic Reflex of Head

This effect refers to an inspiration or gasp resulting from a sudden increase in intratracheal pressure. It is caused by a tracheal vagal afferent reflex into the respiratory center.

▼ CONCLUSION

We have discussed the control of breathing in three major categories:

1. Breathing rate to tidal volume relationship, a balance between airway resistance and lung compliance designed to minimize the work of breathing
2. Chemical control of breathing, designed to regulate the amount of breathing required to satisfy the metabolic needs of the body for CO_2 removal and O_2 consumption
3. Neuronal control of breathing, designed to provide a smooth and rhythmic breathing pattern, also improving effectiveness and reducing the work of breathing

The overall result should be maximization of breathing efficiency. In other words, work expenditure should never exceed ventilatory demands. At a cellular level, the amount of O_2 consumed and CO_2 produced must be matched by the amount being exchanged in the lungs. This must be accomplished as efficiently as possible or it becomes self-defeating.

Many of the abnormal breathing patterns were described as an introduction to the numerous findings concerning lung volumes and capacities encountered in clinical practice. When the mechanisms of breathing are well understood, abnormal breathing patterns can be recognized and more effectively treated.

❖ Review Questions

1. Normal thoracic compliance, expressed in L/cm H_2O, is between
   a. 0.01 and 0.02.
   b. 0.1 and 0.2.
   c. 0.3 and 4.0.
   d. 0.5 and 0.7.
   e. 0.5 and 1.0.
2. Normal airway resistance, measured in cm H_2O/L/sec, is between
   a. 1 and 2.
   b. 2 and 4.
   c. 4 and 6.
   d. 5 and 8.
   e. 5 and 10.
3. How would an increase in airway resistance affect the respiratory rate (RR)/tidal volume (V_T) relationship?

    a. No change in either
    b. Increased V_T and decreased RR
    c. Decreased V_T and RR
    d. Decreased V_T and increased RR
    e. Increased V_T and increased RR
4. Which of the following factors increases the work of breathing?
    i. Increased airway resistance
    ii. Decreased lung compliance
    iii. Decreased chest wall compliance
    iv. Bronchial constriction
    v. Alveolar consolidation

    a. i, ii, iii
    b. ii, iii, iv
    c. iii, iv, v
    d. ii, iii, iv, v
    e. All of the above
5. Given the following variables, determine the inspiratory flow in L\sec:
    P_{Mouth} = 0 cm H_2O
    $P_{Alveolar}$ – -5 cm H_2O
    P_{AW} (airway resistance) = 3.5 cm H_2O/L/sec
    a. 0.25
    b. 0.5
    c. 1.0
    d. 1.5
    e. 3.0
6. The term used to describe the difference in inspiratory and expiratory pressure volume curves is
    a. occipital differential.
    b. pellucidum variance.
    c. hysteresis.
    d. hypophysis.
    e. functional practicum.
7. Spontaneous ventilation is increased when
    a. $[H^+]$ is decreased.
    b. PaO_2 is increased.
    c. CO_2 production is decreased.
    d. O_2 consumption is decreased.
    e. the work of breathing is increased.
8. The central chemoreceptors respond primarily to
    a. CSF $[H^+]$.
    b. $PaCO_2$.
    c. $PvCO_2$.
    d. plasma $[H^+]$.
    e. PaO_2.

9. The peripheral chemoreceptors respond primarily to
   a. $PaCO_2$.
   b. $PvCO_2$.
   c. PaO_2.
   d. $[H^+]$.
   e. pH.

4

LUNG VOLUMES AND GAS FLOW

OBJECTIVES

1. Identify the lung volumes and capacities.

2. Differentiate between restrictive and obstructive lung disorders.

Matthews LR: CARDIOPULMONARY ANATOMY AND PHYSIOLOGY. © 1996 Lippincott–Raven Publishers.

3. Describe deadspace and gas distribution in the lung.

4. Distinguish the factors influencing anatomical deadspace from those influencing alveolar deadspace.

5. Explain the exhaled CO_2 curve.

6. Characterize mixed and end-tidal CO_2 measurements.

7. Define the relationship between $PaCO_2$ and $P_{ET}CO_2$.

8. Describe airway caliber and resistance in terms of tube length and radius.

9. Discuss the impact that gas viscosity has on gas movement.

10. Differentiate laminar flow from turbulent gas flow.

11. Identify the variations in airway resistance from the trachea to the terminal bronchioles.

12. Characterize the regional distribution of gas throughout the lung.

13. State the concept of equal pressure points.

14. Detail the forced expiratory maneuvers.

15. Explain an expiratory flow curve.

16. Explain a flow volume curve.

17. Contrast and compare normal and abnormal breath sounds.

A normal lung has reserves in both inspiratory and expiratory gas volumes. These reserves enable us to expire gas at the end of a normal exhalation and inspire gas at the end of a normal inspiration. Because lung diseases tend to change the relationship of these lung volumes, measurements of these relationships, followed by analysis, can be helpful in diagnosis. This section describes the various lung volumes and their interrelationships.

▼ LUNG VOLUMES AND CAPACITIES

The lung volumes shown in Figure 4-1 are categorized into four distinct types:

1. Tidal volumes (V_T)
2. Inspiratory reserve volume (IRV)
3. Expiratory reserve volume (ERV)
4. Residual volume (RV)

When more than one volume is discussed, the term *capacity* is used. The four capacities are

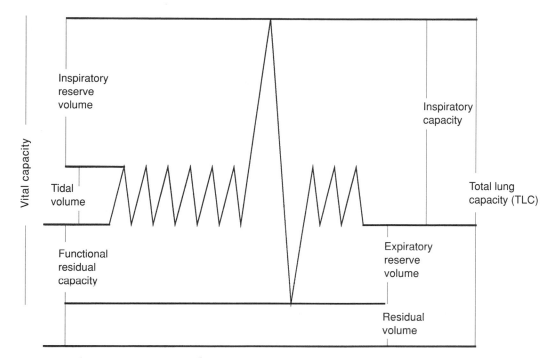

Figure 4-1. Various lung volumes in relationship to total lung capacity.

1. vital capacity (VC)
2. functional residual capacity (FRC)
3. inspiratory capacity (IC)
4. total lung capacity (TLC)

Lung Volumes

V_T is the volume of gas inspired and expired with each normal breath (400–600 mL in a normal, healthy adult), depending on lung and chest wall compliance. **IRV** is the maximum volume of gas that can be inhaled after the end of a normal spontaneous inspiration (normally 2,500–3,500 mL). **ERV** is the maximum amount of volume of gas that can be exhaled after the end of a normal spontaneous expiration (900–1,300 mL in a normal, healthy adult). **RV** is the volume of gas remaining in the lungs after a maximum expiration (normally 1,000–1,400 mL).

Lung Capacities

VC is the maximum volume of gas that can be exhaled after the deepest possible inspiration (range 4,000–5,000 mL in a normal, healthy adult). VC is calculated as

$$VC = IRV + V_T + ERV$$

FRC is the amount of air remaining in the lungs at the end of a normal expiration, and is calculated as

$$FRC = ERV + RV$$

IC is the maximum volume of gas that can be inhaled after normal exhalation of a V_T (normally 3,000–4,000 mL). It is calculated as

$$IC = IRV + V_T$$

TLC is the volume of gas contained in the lungs after maximum inhalation (5,000–6,000 mL in a normal, healthy adult). TLC is calculated as

$$TLC = IRV + ERV + V_T + RV$$

Significance of Lung Volumes and Capacities

Alterations in lung volumes and capacities are indicative of disease processes. The results of tests designed to measure lung volumes allow the clinician to document and quantify the disease's impact on the lung. If lung and chest wall compliance change or tissue destruction results in air being trapped in the lung, the relative size of lung volume changes.

Two primary alterations have been described: restrictive and obstructive. **Restrictive alterations** involve an overall decrease in total lung capacities and volumes with relatively unchanged relationships between IRV, ERV, and V_T. Diseases that typically result in restricted lung volumes include those that affect the chest wall (e.g., kyphoscoliosis, neuromuscular weakness, and obesity) and

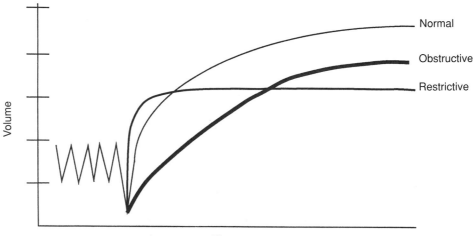

Figure 4-2.   The difference between expiratory flow curves in obstructive and restrictive lung disease.

those that affect the lung (e.g., sarcoidosis, asbestosis causing lung fibrosis, and pneumonia).

These diseases result in a decreased lung compliance, reducing overall lung volume or increasing the force of elastic recoil in lung tissue.

Obstructive alterations involve an overall increase in TLC with decreased IRV, ERV, and V_T. Emphysema and asthma are diseases that typically result in obstructive lung disease (Figure 4-2).

▼ DEADSPACE VENTILATION

Deadspace

Deadspace refers to the volume of gas in the airways and the lungs that does not take part in gas exchange. It is important to consider because, although it plays no role in gas exchange, it still requires work to move this volume into and out of the lungs. If a disease results in an increase in deadspace, then the wasted work is increased, contributing to a less efficient ventilation system. There are two types of deadspace, **anatomical** and **alveolar**, collectively referred to as **physiological deadspace**:

Physiological deadspace — Anatomical deadspace + Alveolar deadspace

Anatomical Deadspace

Anatomical deadspace is the total volume of gases contained in the airways from the mouth or nose down to the alveoli. This volume in normal, healthy individuals is approximately 2 mL/kg (1 mL/lb) of ideal body weight. It also can be estimated based on body height. Anatomical deadspace can be affected by age, airway positioning, bronchial smooth muscle tone, and transpulmonary pressures. (See Chapter 2 for a listing of the transpulmonary pressures necessary to effect ventilation.)

A small increase in anatomical deadspace occurs with age. It may be the result of lost elastic lung fiber with a greater than normal increase in connecting airway volume as the lung is stretched open during inspiration.

Airway position can increase or decrease deadspace by either stretching out or compressing the upper airway. When the neck is extended and the jaw is pushed forward, deadspace can be increased. With the neck and chin depressed, deadspace can actually be decreased.

Bronchial smooth muscle tone can have an impact on anatomical deadspace by physically changing the space contained in the air passageways. Constricted airway smooth muscle results in a reduction in deadspace, and relaxed airway smooth muscle results in an increase in deadspace. The reduced work of breathing associated with bronchodilation (smooth muscle relaxation) overrides the problem associated with an increase in deadspace.

Transpulmonary pressure can either pull out the airways, a result of lateral traction caused by an inspiratory effort, or compress the airways with pressure, something that can occur during forced expiration.

Posture not only affects lung volumes, but also impacts on anatomical deadspace. Simply changing position, for example, from a sitting to a supine position, can reduce anatomical deadspace by as much as 30%.

Alveolar Deadspace

Alveolar deadspace is the volume of inspired gas that reaches an alveolus but does not take part in gas exchange. This is a result of absent or inadequate blood supply into the capillary bed. In normal, healthy individuals this volume is too small to be accurately measured. However, if disease results in diminished blood flow from hypotension, decreased cardiac output, or pulmonary embolism, alveolar deadspace can be increased. This results because ventilation is in excess of perfusion, which is defined as supplying an organ or tissue with oxygen (O_2) and necessary nutrients.

Alveolar deadspace should be differentiated from the deadspace effect. Alveolar deadspace is the absence of blood supply to an alveolus, whereas the deadspace effect refers to reduced or diminished blood supply.

Deadspace Determination

In healthy individuals deadspace accounts for approximately one third of the V_T. Determination of the relative relationship between the volume of deadspace and the size of the V_T can be calculated using the following formula:

Physiologic $V_D/V_T = [PaCO_2 - P\overline{E}CO_2]/PaCO_2$
    (deadspace-to-tidal-volume ratio is expressed as a decimal)

where V_D is the volume of deadspace; V_T is the tidal volume; $PaCO_2$ is the partial pressure of carbon dioxide (CO_2) in arterial blood, which is determined by analyzing a sample of arterial blood taken from the patient; and $P\overline{E}CO_2$ is the mixed expired PCO_2, measured using an analyzer after collecting exhaled gas in a large bag (Douglas bag). This last value is the average concentration of CO_2 collected for at least 3 minutes. Continuous flushing is also necessary to be sure all original gas in the system is removed (see Clinical Applications Box 4-1).

Technique for Determination: How it Works

Because CO_2 diffuses so readily between the blood and the alveoli when blood and alveolar gas are matched, CO_2 in both compartments is essentially equal

---

Clinical Applications Box 4-1   Using a Douglas Bag

Continuous flushing allows any residual gas in the bag to flow out through a continuous leak as it fills with gas expired by the patient. This is done to ensure that any gas that is then measured comes from the patient and not the bag. This technique also ensures that all gas that was originally in the system has been removed.

in partial pressure. As a result, we analyze arterial CO_2 ($PaCO_2$) and assume it is the same as alveolar CO_2 ($PACO_2$). $PaCO_2$ is similar or equal to $PACO_2$. $P\overline{E}CO_2$ is a measurement of the average concentration of CO_2 exhaled and includes gas exchange and non–gas exchange volume in the lungs and airways. Therefore, the difference between $PaCO_2$ and $P\overline{E}CO_2$ can be indicative of the volume of gas not taking part in gas exchange. This situation is expressed mathematically as follows:

$$V_D/V_T = PaCO_2 - P\overline{E}CO_2/PaCO_2$$

If there were no gas exchange units in the lungs, then $P\overline{E}CO_2$ would contain no CO_2. (For our purposes, air has such a low concentration of CO_2, we consider it to be absent.)

$$PaCO_2 \text{ (normal value)} = 40 \text{ mmHg}$$
$$P\overline{E}CO_2 = 0 \text{ mmHg}$$

Therefore,

$$V_D/V_T = 40 - 0/40$$
$$= 1$$

To convert to a percentage, we multiply by 100. Thus, the deadspace percentage in relationship to the size of the V_T is 100%.

If we did not require connecting airways and all of the gas inhaled were to take part in gas exchange, then our exhaled gas would be derived entirely from functional gas exchange units. Thus, $PaCO_2$ would equal $P\overline{E}CO_2$ and all exhaled gas would have the same concentration of CO_2. Therefore,

$$V_D/V_T = 40 - 40/40$$
$$= 0 \times 100$$
$$= 0\%$$

Under normal circumstances, exhaled gas is a combination of alveolar gas and deadspace gas (from connecting airways and poorly perfused gas exchange units). Therefore, the concentration of exhaled CO_2 from alveolar gas exchange units is diluted with air containing no CO_2. This lowers the $P\overline{E}CO_2$ value. If a normal V_T is 500 mL in a 75 kg male, he would have approximately 150 mL (2×75) of deadspace. (Anatomical deadspace is approximately 2 mL/kg ideal body weight.) Therefore,

$$V_D/V_T = 150 \text{ mL}/500 \text{ mL}$$
$$= 0.30$$
$$= 30\%$$

If we use the same method that was used previously, we would see that 150 mL of exhaled gas has no CO_2 in it and 350 mL ($500 - 150$) has an alveolar gas concentration. When added together

1. 70% of the V_T has a PCO_2 OF 40. Therefore, $0.7 \times 40 = 28$.
2. 30% of the V_T has no CO_2. Therefore, $0.3 \times 0 = 0$.

When the two concentrations are added together, $0 + 28 = 28$ mmHg (concentration of exhaled gas). Therefore,

V_D/V_T = [normal $PaCO_2$ − mixed exhaled CO_2]/40 (normal $PaCO_2$), or
= [40 − 28]/40
= 12/40
= 0.3
= 30% (in a healthy 75-kg male).

It can be seen that this dilution calculation can be used to approximate deadspace volume to V_T relationships. Remember, however, that the clinical relevance of these calculations is dependent on a stable V_T.

Deadspace volume also can be calculated using the following formula:

$$V_D = [V_T \times (PaCO_2 - P\overline{E}CO_2)]/PaCO_2$$

This volume will be the total volume of deadspace, both anatomical and alveolar. Anatomical deadspace volume can be calculated using the following formula:

$$\text{Anatomical } V_D = [P_{ET}CO_2 - P\overline{E}CO_2]/P_{ET}CO_2 \times V_T$$

where $P_{ET}CO_2$ is the average concentration of end tidal CO_2.

In normal, healthy individuals there is little or no alveolar deadspace; therefore, physiological deadspace and anatomical deadspace are equal. This means that $PaCO_2$ is approximately equal to $P_{ET}CO_2$ (Figure 4-3).

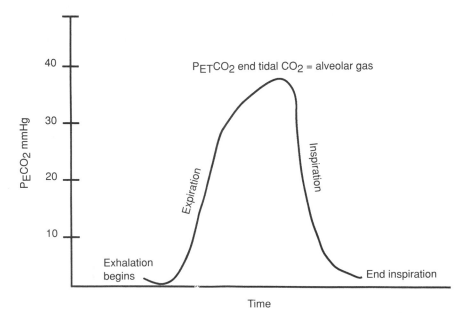

Figure 4-3. The level of CO_2 being measured at the patient's mouth continuously throughout the breathing cycle.

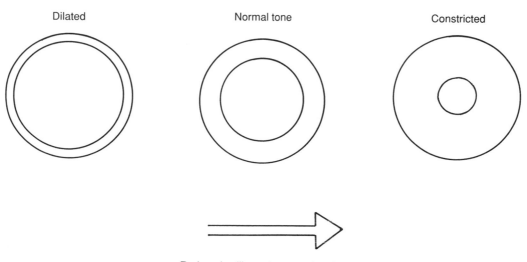

Figure 4-4. **The effect of airway caliber on the resistance to gas flow.**

Concentration of CO_2 is measured from the beginning to the end of an exhalation. The concentration will go from zero to alveolar concentration (Figure 4-4). This, of course, is for a normal, healthy individual at rest. As end-expired or end-tidal CO_2 increases, it is an indication that alveolar deadspace is reducing in size and vice versa.

Example #1

If there is no deadspace (possible for fish but not humans), the average CO_2 concentration and the end-tidal CO_2 concentration would be equal. When $P_{ET}CO_2 = P_{\overline{E}}CO_2$,

$$P_{ET}CO_2 = 40 \text{ mmHg}$$
$$P_{\overline{E}}CO_2 = 40 \text{ mmHg}$$
$$V_T = 500 \text{ mL}$$
$$\text{Anatomical } V_D = V_T \times [(P_{ET}CO_2 - P_{\overline{E}}CO_2)/P_{ET}CO_2]$$
$$= 500 \times ([40 - 40]/40)$$
$$= 500 \times 0$$
$$= 0$$

Example #2

If anatomical deadspace is normal, then $P_{ET}CO_2$ will still equal 40 mmHg. However, the average measurement of $P_{\overline{E}}CO_2$ will contain exhaled gas that has essentially no CO_2. This reduces the average value to a concentration indicative of the volume of anatomical deadspace:

$$P_{ET}CO_2 = 40 \text{ mmHg}$$
$$P_{\overline{E}}CO_2 = 28 \text{ mmHg}$$
$$V_T = 500 \text{ mL}$$
$$\text{Anatomical } V_D = V_T \times ([P_{ET}CO_2 - P_{\overline{E}}CO_2]/P_{ET}CO_2)$$
$$= 500 \times ([40 - 28]/40)$$
$$= 500 \times 0.3$$
$$= 150 \text{ mL}$$

As alveolar deadspace increases, $P_{ET}CO_2$ and $P_{\overline{E}}CO_2$ decrease proportionally, thus not have a significant impact on the accuracy of this calculation.

$$\text{Alveolar deadspace} = \text{Physiological deadspace} - \text{Anatomical deadspace}$$

The physiological deadspace volume or V_T relationship includes both the anatomical deadspace and the alveolar deadspace. For this reason, subtracting anatomical deadspace from the physiological deadspace provides a good indication of the amount of alveolar deadspace.

$PaCO_2/P_{ET}CO_2$ Difference

Using an end-tidal CO_2 monitor to approximate alveolar deadspace is a simple and convenient method of assessing changes in alveolar deadspace. As alveolar deadspace increases, $P_{ET}CO_2$ decreases. Remember that $P_{ET}CO_2$ will always be lower than $PaCO_2$ because of exhaled gas mixing. However, it can be an indicator of the ongoing magnitude of alveolar deadspace (Figure 4-3).

The following equation can be used to compute alveolar deadspace:

$$\text{Alveolar deadspace} = [PaCO_2 - P_{ET}CO_2]/PaCO_2$$

Physiological Impact of Increased Deadspace

If deadspace volume increases, minute volume (MV) must increase to maintain the volume of alveolar ventilation.

Example #3

$$MV = 5 \text{ L}$$
$$V_D/V_T = 0.3$$
$$\text{Alveolar ventilation} = MV \times 0.7$$
$$= 3.5 \text{ Lpm}$$
$$\text{Deadspace ventilation} = MV \times 0.3$$
$$= 1.5 \text{ Lpm}$$

The alveolar ventilation must be maintained even with an increased deadspace. Therefore, if the deadspace increased to 0.5, minute ventilation would increase as follows:

$$V_D/V_T = 0.5$$
$$\text{Alveolar ventilation} = 3.5 \text{ Lpm}$$
$$\text{Required MV} = [\text{Alveolar ventilation}]/V_D/V_T$$
$$= 3.5/0.5$$
$$= 7.5 \text{ L}$$

Therefore, in order to maintain the required alveolar ventilation when V_D/V_T is increased to 0.5, minute ventilation must be increased to 7.5 Lpm.

Effect of Changing Tidal Volume

If the V_T is 500 mL and V_D/V_T is 0.3, the alveolar ventilation and deadspace for a given V_T are calculated as follows:

$$\text{Alveolar ventilation} = 500 \times 0.7 \text{ mL} = 350 \text{ mL}$$

$$\text{Deadspace ventilation} = 500 \times 0.3 \text{ mL}$$

$$= 150 \text{ mL}$$

If the V_T is reduced to 300 mL, deadspace volume remains the same but V_D/V_T increases to 0.5. This is because, regardless of the size of the V_T, anatomical deadspace remains the same. Therefore, in order to maintain alveolar ventilation, the individual would need to increase the number of tidal volumes per minute. This means increased minute ventilation and increased energy expenditure for breathing.

▼ AIRWAY CALIBER AND RESISTANCE

An increase in airway resistance is inversely related to airway caliber. That is to say, the smaller the caliber of the airway, the more work is required to move the gas. In fact, the work of breathing required to move gas increases exponentially as the airway shrinks in diameter.

Poiseuille's equation describes the basic factors that determine the resistance to flow in terms of the following:

1. Length of the tube, or airway (l)
2. Viscosity of the flowing substance (n)
3. Radius of the tube (r)

Because the length of the tube and the viscosity of the gas do not vary in a given individual as long as a flow is laminar (smooth and uniform), the most important factor becomes airway radius. A decrease in radius by 50% (vascular or bronchial) causes a 16-fold increase in the resistance to flow (Figure 4-4).

The work needed to maintain laminar flow at a given rate is much lower than that required to accommodate turbulent flow. Turbulence can be created by sudden direction changes and high-velocity flow, narrowed airways, or pressurized gas. Turbulent flow occurs most commonly in the larger airways (trachea, bronchi), where flow is highest.

When flow is turbulent, gas viscosity becomes the single most important determinant of whether ventilation is disrupted. If turbulence becomes a significant problem, a helium–O_2 gas mixture can be administered to the patient. Because this gas compound has a lower viscosity and total weight than does the nitrogen–O_2 mixture normally breathed, it is more easily inspired and expired, thereby reducing the work of breathing until the underlying disease can be ameliorated.

Airway Caliber

A number of factors affect airway caliber, some by increasing it and others by decreasing it (Table 4-1).

Bronchodilation refers to expansion of the bronchial passages and is always associated with a reduction in airway resistance. Bronchodilation is achieved in any one of the following ways:

1. Inhaling deeply: inspiration exerts radial traction that pulls the airways out, a condition that increases their diameters
2. Hypoxia and hypercapnia (increased CO_2 in inspired gas)
3. Discharge of epinephrine from the adrenal medulla
4. Beta-adrenergic therapy
5. Any neuronal chemical mediator that results in increased levels of cyclic adenosine monophosphate (cAMP)

Bronchoconstriction, on the other hand, functions by reducing airway diameter and increasing airway resistance. It, too, results from any of a number of causative conditions:

1. Expiration: the pressure applied externally to the airways in the course of normal expiration makes this a natural means of effecting bronchoconstriction.
2. Laryngeal irritation: laryngeal irritation may result in laryngospasm, constricting the airway and therefore increasing airway resistance.
3. Vagal stimulation through subepithelial nerve fibers is a reflex arc that causes the cough.
4. Mast cell degranulation and subsequent release of chemical mediators: the immediate results are bronchospasm, edema, and increased mucus production (see Chapter 15). Asthmatic patients are hypersensitive to laryngeal irritation and mast cell degranulation, making them more susceptible to airway constriction and increased work of breathing.

TABLE 4-1   Bronchodilators and Bronchoconstrictors

Bronchodilators	Bronchoconstrictors
Taking a deep breath	Expiration
Hypoxia and hypercapnia	Laryngeal irritation
Discharge of epinephrine from the adrenal medulla	Vagal stimulation through subepithelial nerve fibers
Beta-adrenergic therapy	Mast cell degranulation and subsequent release of chemical mediators
Any neuronal chemical mediator that results in increased levels of cyclic AMP	Beta-adrenergic blockade therapy

5. Beta-adrenergic blockade therapy: this therapy can result in bronchospasm, and thus bronchoconstriction.

The level of airway sensitivity varies greatly from one individual to another. Hypersensitive airways are present in some individuals, a condition commonly referred to as asthma. In any case, increased airway resistance results in a reduction in the ability to move fresh gas into the lungs and remove gas containing CO_2. The muscles of ventilation will also produce more CO_2 and consume more O_2.

▼ DISTRIBUTION OF VENTILATION

Even in normal, healthy individuals, the movement of air into and out of the lungs is unevenly distributed as a result of

1. regional differences in lung volume change during inspiration
2. diaphragmatic effects on lung expansion
3. gravitational effects on lung expansion
4. variations in airway resistance and lung compliance

Regional Differences in Lung Volume Changes During Inspiration

These differences affect the amount of gas entering a region of the lung. Remember that the size of a given V_T is determined by the extent of change in intrathoracic volume. Because the lung and thorax are of nonuniform shape, inspiration affects the volumes of the upper and lower portions differently: the lower part changes more. Also, during the inspiratory phase, as the chest wall is pulled out and the diaphragm is pulled down, the outer portion of the lung is stretched more than the inner portion. Therefore, comparatively speaking, the peripheral regions of the lungs are expanded to a greater degree than are the deeper, more internal regions.

If gas distribution is monitored for RV up to TLC, the first gas entering the lung will go to the apex (in an upright subject) and then it will gradually be distributed into the base of the lung. However, it is important to realize that the largest overall volume distribution will be into the base.

Diaphragmatic Effects on Lung Expansion

When the diaphragm contracts and pulls down on the lung, movement of the lung is more pronounced in the bases than in the apex. Also, the lung is, in some respects, anchored to the *hilum*, the area through which the venous and arterial blood supplies and the lymphatics enter the lung. As a result, any downward movement will be less effective on lung regions above this area.

Gravitational Effects on Lung Expansion

In an upright position, the weight of the lung pulling downward tends to stretch out the upper portions of the lung. This is one of the reasons that gas movement enters the apex of the lung first, after a maximum exhalation maneuver is performed.

Variations in Airway Resistance and Lung Compliance

Because diseases rarely affect the lung in a uniform manner, it is not uncommon to see a combination of diseased and healthy tissue. If airway resistance is nonuniform, gas distribution will also be nonuniform. The same principle applies to compliance in terms of lung expansion. Variations in lung compliance will lead to variations in lung expansion during inspiration. In normal, healthy lung tissue, the effect of gravity and lung weight on compliance as well as their effect on lateral traction of airways accounts for the vertical nonuniformity of the distribution of ventilation.

▼ EQUILIBRATION OF PRESSURE THROUGHOUT THE LUNG

Combining the effects of both resistance and compliance produces a relationship that can predict how quickly a region will fill with gas. For a given pressure difference across a given set of airways, as resistance increases (airway narrows), the flow into the region decreases. This means gas flow into this area will be reduced. As a result, the area will expand slower than areas with lower airway resistance. If compliance is reduced (the lung becomes stiff) for a given pressure difference across the airways, volume will be reduced. This means if a region of the lung is less compliant than another, it will receive less volume.

Inspiratory Time and Time Constants

For a given inspiratory time, variations in compliance and resistance will result in uneven gas distribution throughout the lung. The time it takes for pressures to equilibrate and gas flow to cease can be described in terms of time constants.

Time constant (seconds) =
$$\text{Compliance (L/cm } H_2O) \times \text{Resistance (cm } H_2O/L/sec)$$

Example #4

With normal compliance and resistance

Time constant (seconds) = 0.1 L/cm H_2O × 1.0 cm H_2O/L/sec
= 0.1 second

Because as the flow of gas moves into a given region pressure rises and the pressure difference is decreased, it takes three time constants for pressure equilibration to occur (95% of equilibration). In this case

three time constants = 3 × 0.1 sec
= 0.3 seconds

If the compliance or resistance increases, the amount of time for equilibration to occur will be increased. The reverse is also true: if resistance or compliance is reduced, the time required for equilibration will be reduced.

Example #5

Increased resistance, normal compliance:

one time constant = 0.1 L/cm H_2O × 6.0 cm H_2O/L/sec
= 0.6 seconds

Resistance is increased sixfold, and the amount of time for equilibration to occur is also increased sixfold. This region fills slowly.

Example #6

Normal resistance, reduced compliance:

one time constant = 0.025 L/cm H_2O × 1.0 cm H_2O/L/sec
= 0.025 seconds

Both compliance and the time required for equilibration to occur are reduced fourfold. This area of greatly reduced compliance develops a small volume quickly, and then the surrounding areas, which are more compliant, continue to expand around it to occupy the space it would have normally occupied.

▼ FLOW VOLUME CURVE MEASUREMENTS OF LUNG FUNCTION

A common method of assessing lung function is by the use of a flow volume curve. The patient is asked to perform a maximum expiratory then maximum inspiratory effort. The flow volume curve generated represents the expiratory/inspiratory flow developed by the patient relative to a given lung volume. Flow is recorded in liters per second and volume is recorded in liters. This measurement can generate an almost unlimited number of measurements throughout the maneuver. The most common expiratory measurements used for interpretation are as follows:

1. Forced vital capacity (FVC)
2. Peak expiratory flow rate (PEFR)
3. Forced expiratory volume at 50% of expired volume (FEF$_{50\%}$ or V$_{max50}$)

These measurements are explained at length below.

The one inspiratory measurement worth mentioning is the peak inspiratory flow rate. This flow can be significantly reduced when an airway obstruction is extrathoracic (occurs in any area from the sternal notch upwards).

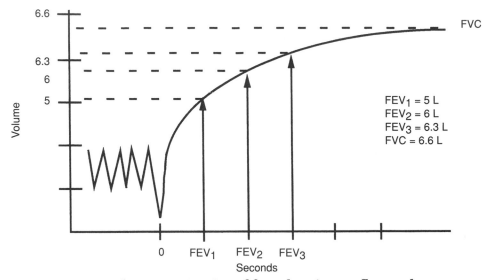

Figure 4-5.   A graphic representation of forced expiratory flow at the beginning of inspiration (200–1,200 mL) and in the middle of exhalation (mid 50%).

Forced Expiratory Flows

Forced Vital Capacity

This is the maximum volume of gas that can be expired as forcefully and rapidly as possible after maximal inspiration. The FVC is normally equal to the ordinary VC. FVC may be less than VC if an obstructive process is present, such as in emphysema.

Flow volume curves also can provide forced expiratory flow in time intervals (i.e., FEV in 1, 2, or 3 seconds) (Figure 4-5). Diagnosis of upper airway, tracheal, or mainstem bronchi abnormalities can be assisted by the characteristic flow limitation at specific FVC levels.

Forced Expiratory Volume (FEV time, or FEV_T)

This measures the volume of gas expired over a given time interval during the performance of an FVC maneuver (Figure 4-6). This can determine the severity of airflow obstruction. A decreased FEV_T may result from airway narrowing due to mucus secretion, bronchospasm, inflammation, or loss of elastic support in lung tissue.

FEV in 1 second (FEV_1) is the most commonly used spirometric measurement to assess airway obstruction. Its validity depends largely on the cooperation of the subject and the expertise of the therapist.

Peak Expiratory Flow Rate

Peak expiratory flow rate reflects the maximum flow of expiratory gas during the forced expiratory maneuver (Figure 4-7). It may be reduced in obstructive

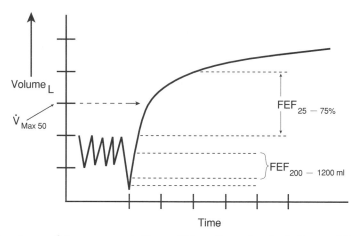

Figure 4-6. A graphic representation of time forced exhalation, with volumes measured at 1, 2, and 3 seconds.

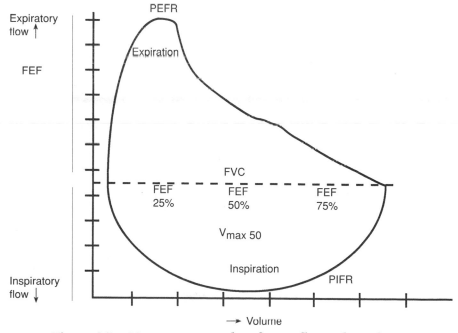

Figure 4-7. Measurements taken from a flow volume loop.

disease processes and normal or even elevated during restrictive disease processes.

Forced Expiratory Flow (FEF$_{50\%}$, or V$_{max50}$)

This is the measured expiratory flow at the point where 50% of the patient's VC has been expelled. This also can be measured at 25% (V$_{max25}$) or 75% (V$_{max75}$) of the expelled VC. A reduction in these values from normal is indicative of obstructive disease.

Maximum Voluntary Ventilation

Maximum voluntary ventilation is the absolute maximum volume that can be breathed over a 10- to 15-second period. This value is converted to liters per minute and can be used to measure ventilatory muscle function or abnormal lung, thorax, or resistance processes. It also can be useful in predicting exercise limitations.

Total Lung Capacity

Total lung capacity, the maximum volume of gas contained in the lungs, can be measured by a number of different techniques beyond the scope of this text. However, it is worth mentioning as a commonly performed test. This value is generally elevated in chronic obstructive pulmonary disease (COPD). The size of the FRC in relationship to the total lung capacity is particularly important.

Equal Pressure Point

During forced expiratory maneuvers, two forces contribute to the generation of alveolar pressure: the pressure derived from the elastic recoil of the lung and the pleural pressure (Figure 4-8). Because the elastic recoil of the lung

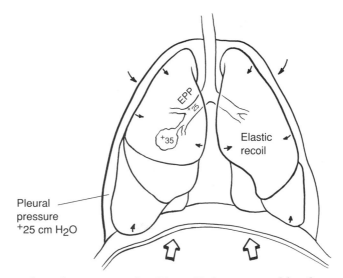

Figure 4-8.   A pleural pressure of +25 cm H$_2$O generated by the muscles of expiration. The pressure generated by elastic recoil is 10 cm H$_2$O.

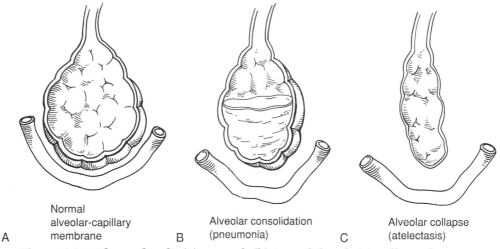

A   Normal
     alveolar-capillary
     membrane   B

     Alveolar consolidation
     (pneumonia)   C

     Alveolar collapse
     (atelectasis)

Figure 4-9.   Three alveoli: (a) normal, (b) consolidated, (c) collapsed.

contributes to the generation of alveolar pressure, the pressure within the air-space is greater than the pressure pushing in from the outside (pleural pressure).

The pressure resulting from elastic recoil gradually decreases, as does airway pressure from the alveolus to the mouth. This means that at some point, pressure inside the airway will be equal to the pressure outside the airway. This point is known as the equal pressure point (EPP), and it exists as the result of the balance between the pressure inside and outside the airway. There comes a point at which pressure inside the airway is less than the pressure outside the airway, a condition that results in airway collapse and increased expiratory resistance. This collapse is, in most cases, impeded by the airway's rigid structure of cartilage and supporting structures. When this happens, greater expiratory effort will not increase expiratory flow because of its effect on reducing the size of the airway (Figure 4-9). This effect is present during forced expiratory maneuvers only and does not occur during quiet breathing. In healthy individuals, EPP occurs only at lung volumes below FRC.

▼ BREATH SOUNDS

Normally, chest sounds heard on auscultation (see Clinical Applications Box 4-2) are that of air rushing through the airways, traveling from the mouth down into the lungs and back out. Because there is a remarkable change in gas flow between the trachea and the alveoli, breath sounds also vary in nature and pitch.

Around the trachea and larger bronchi, the sound is loud and high pitched. These sounds are commonly referred to as **bronchial breath sounds**

Clinical Applications Box 4-2   Auscultation

Auscultation is a term used to describe audible assessment of the chest. It is performed by using a stethoscope to obtain information about the flow of gas through the tracheobronchial tree. Auscultation can be helpful in the identification of

1. alveolar consolidation, which occurs when the alveoli are full of fluid or secretions instead of air (Figure 4-9)
2. excess secretions or fluid accumulation
3. bronchial obstruction
4. bronchospasm
5. proper airway placement

Proper auscultation involves placing the stethoscope from one side of the chest to the other from top to bottom. Each area is listened to while the patient inhales and exhales at an increased rate and depth of breathing.

---

and are more evident during expiration. Further down in the chest, over the lungs, breath sounds are softer and lower pitched. These sounds are more evident during inspiration and are commonly referred to as bronchovesicular, or vesicular, sounds. Having the patient take a deep breath and then exhale passively can accentuate these breath sounds, making them easier to interpret. Abnormalities may be indicative of an underlying disease process or trauma.

Abnormal Breath Sounds

Bronchial breath sounds heard over lung tissue (a parenchymal area) are abnormal and result from sound being transmitted through consolidated regions of the lung. Remember that liquid transmits sound more readily than does air. Diseases causing alveolar collapse or consolidation produce a bronchial type of sound over the affected area of the lung.

A **pneumothorax** (gas or air in the lung) or hypoventilation (reduced rate and depth of breathing) results in diminished breath sounds because of the increased airspace or reduction in gas movement.

Crackles, also known as rales, are a result of fluid in the small to medium-sized airways. As gas moves back and forth through this area, a crackling sound is produced. It is similar in sound to crushing cellophane. This is typically heard during inspiration (often used to describe inspiratory and expiratory secretion sounds).

Rhonchi are coarse sounds heard during expiration. They result from secretions in the larger airways and are often absent after a cough.

Wheezing is a sound produced by bronchospasm. It exists in all bronchospastic disorders and is a cardinal finding in bronchial asthma. These sounds are high pitched and whistling in nature, lasting throughout expiration.

Pleural friction rub is a result of inflamed pleural membranes. The normal smooth movement between the parietal and visceral pleura is resisted. This creates a characteristic sound, creaking in nature, often over an area where the patient complains of pain. (See Glossary for a complete description of individual breath sounds.)

▼ CONCLUSION

Because effective gas exchange in the lung depends on patent airways (those through which it is easy to breathe), much of a therapist's time is spent keeping the airways open and clear of excess fluid or mucus. Overall regional lung volumes also can be affected by airway patency. A comprehensive understanding of the normal gas movement in the lung and the resulting volumes is an important prerequisite to understanding the changes brought on by disease. Because lung disease causes bronchoconstriction, swelling of the airways, and alveolar consolidation, breathing may become difficult, if not impossible. The effectiveness of treatment and the modifications necessary can only be recognized if the underlying physiological processes are well understood.

❖ Review Questions

1. Functional residual capacity (FRC) is a combination of
   a. ERV + RV.
   b. IRV + V_T.
   c. IRV + ERV + V_T.
   d. IRV + ERV + RV
   e. IRV + ERV + V_T + RV.
2. Restrictive lung disease may be a result of
   i. kyphoscoliosis.
   ii. sarcoidosis.
   iii. asbestosis.
   iv. COPD.
   v. pneumonia.

   a. i, ii, iii
   b. ii, iii, iv
   c. iii, iv, v
   d. i, ii, iii, v
   e. All of the above
3. The resistance to flow may be affected by
   i. the length of the tube.
   ii. chest wall rigidity.
   iii. the viscosity of the flowing substance.
   iv. lung compliance.
   v. the radius of the tube.

   a. i, ii, iii
   b. ii, iii, iv
   c. i, iii, v
   d. iii, iv, v
   e. All of the above
4. Airway resistance is highest in the
   a. trachea.
   b. pharynx
   c. segmental bronchi.
   d. terminal bronchioles.
   e. alveolar ducts.
5. Which of the following factors causes airway dilation?
   i.   Hypoxia
   ii. Hypercapnia
   iii. Epinephrine
   iv. Beta-adrenergic stimulation
   v.   Increased levels of cyclic AMP

   a. i, ii, iii
   b. ii, iii, iv
   c. i, iii, v
   d. iii, iv, v
   e. All of the above
6. Anatomical deadspace may be affected by
   i.   age.
   ii. airway position.
   iii. bronchial smooth muscle tone.
   iv. posture.
   v.   alveolar consolidation.

   a. i, ii, iii
   b. ii, iii, iv
   c. ii, iii, v
   d. i, ii, iii, iv
   e. All of the above

   Given the following information, calculate the deadspace volumes for
   Questions 7–10:

$$V_T = 1,000 \text{ mL}$$
$$PaCO_2 = 40 \text{ mmHg}$$
$$PvCO_2 = 46 \text{ mmHg}$$
$$PaO_2 = 80 \text{ mmHg}$$
$$P\bar{E}CO_2 = 27 \text{ mmHg}$$
$$P_{ET}CO_2 = 38 \text{ mmHg}$$

7. The alveolar deadspace is
   a. 36 mL.
   b. 130 mL.
   c. 173 mL.

    d. 325 mL.

    e. 375 mL.

8. The anatomical deadspace volume is

    a. 36 mL.

    b. 130 mL.

    c. 173 mL.

    d. 289 mL.

    e. 750 mL.

9. The physiological deadspace volume is

    a. 36 mL.

    b. 130 mL.

    c. 325 mL.

    d. 425 mL.

    e. 513 mL.

10. Calculate one time constant using the following information.

        Compliance $= 0.05$ L/cm H_2O

        Resistance $= 3$ cm H_2O/L/sec

    Alveolar pressure $- 3$ cm H_2O

          $P_M = 0$ cm H_2O

    a. 0.15 seconds

    b. 0.30 seconds

    c. 0.45 seconds

    d. 0.60 seconds

    c. 0.75 seconds

5

MAINTAINING FUNCTIONAL RESIDUAL CAPACITY

OBJECTIVES

1. Discuss the concept of lung volume maintenance.

2. Describe the pleura.

3. Characterize the movement of fluid through the pleura and discuss pleural fluid testing.

4. Distinguish transudative from exudative pleural effusions.

5. List the factors affecting the alveolar gas concentrations of oxygen and carbon dioxide.

6. Express the alveolar air equation.

7. Explain the importance of the sigh mechanism.

8. Characterize surfactant as it is conceptualized in both the wet and dry lung models.

Matthews LR: CARDIOPULMONARY ANATOMY AND PHYSIOLOGY. © 1996 Lippincott–Raven Publishers.

9. Express Hooke's law.

The lungs remain inflated to maintain a functional residual capacity (FRC) at all times despite the fact that alveolar pressure is zero relative to atmospheric pressure. A number of complex dynamic factors interact to establish this delicate balance.

The lung is attached to the chest wall by the *visceral pleura*. It is held firmly up against the *parietal pleura* and any movement of the chest wall, in or out, is transmitted to the lung. This attachment cannot be explained in terms of cohesive or adhesive forces. The lungs are continuously pulling in because of their elastic tendency to collapse. The chest wall is a semi-rigid structure that holds the lungs open. The combination of the lung pulling in and the chest wall holding the lung open results in a balance (Figure 5-1a).

The position of the tidal volume (V_T) relative to FRC and inspiratory reserve volume (IRV) is a result of these two forces working against each other.

This chapter describes the factors responsible for maintaining an appropriate lung volume:

1. The pleura
2. Alveolar gas concentration
3. Surfactant
4. Parenchymal elasticity

▼ CHEST WALL–LUNG BALANCE

If compliance increases due to loss of elastic fiber (such as in emphysema), the chest wall can pull the lung out (Figure 5-1b). This increases FRC and decreases inspiratory capacity (IC) as the V_T nears the maximum lung volume. In contrast, if the compliance decreases (such as in fibrosis), the lung will pull the chest wall in, reducing FRC and possibly the IC as well (Figure 5-1c).

The lung must remain in a partially inflated state at all times for breathing to require a minimal energy expenditure and for gas exchange to occur continuously. The first breath of life requires a major energy expenditure (40–60 cm H_2O), but once the lungs are inflated, only minimal effort is required for breathing. This maintenance of lung volumes is essential if the work of breathing is to be minimized.

▼ THE PLEURA

Maintenance of the Potential Space

The potential, or pleural, space refers to the area between the visceral and parietal pleurae. Except for a small amount of viscous fluid that lubricates this potential space, it is essentially empty. The lubricant found in this area is actu-

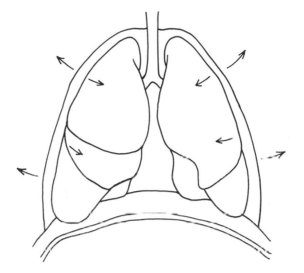

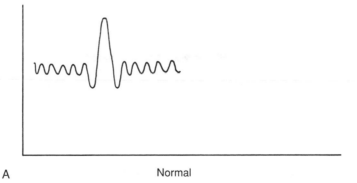

A   Normal

Figure 5-1.   The relationship between compliance and lung volume. (a) A normal compliance–lung volume relationship. (b) A reduction in lung volume caused by a reduction in lung compliance. (c) Increased lung compliance can move the tidal volume closer to total lung capacity.

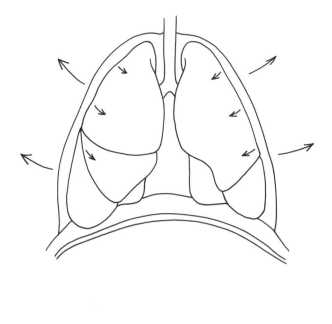

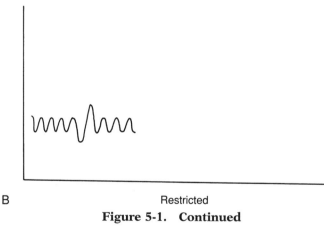

B   Restricted

Figure 5-1.   Continued

ally a surface active agent (*surfactant*). This fluid can reduce the coefficient of friction by 90%. When the chest wall and diaphragm are moving (creating lung expansion and deflation) there must be free, almost frictionless movement. Fluid must not accumulate in this area because it will actually encroach on space normally occupied by lung tissue. The most common cause for accumulation of fluid in this space is infection. White blood cells and other infectious matter plug up the lymphatics (see Chapter 12) and cause (1) a buildup of protein and (2) an increase in colloidal osmotic pressure, resulting in failure of fluid reabsorption (**pleural effusion**). (Normally, the visceral pleura and the lung absorb a considerable amount of fluid.)

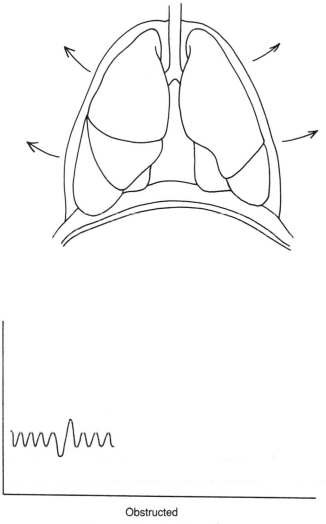

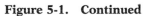

C   Obstructed

Figure 5-1.   Continued

The parietal pleura is a smooth, semitransparent mesothelial membrane that lines the thoracic cavity. It receives its circulatory support from the systemic vasculature. The hydrostatic pressure (blood pressure) in the systemic capillaries is approximately $+30$ cm H_2O. The systemic oncotic pressure (osmotic pressure) is -34 cm H_2O. This results in a net pull of fluid into the systemic capillaries of 4 cm H_2O. However, pleural space hydrostatic pressure is -5 cm H_2O, as is oncotic pressure. The combined negative pressure results in fluid movement into the potential space (Figure 5-2).

The visceral pleura is also a smooth semitransparent mesothelial membrane. It lines the lungs and receives its circulatory support from the pulmonary

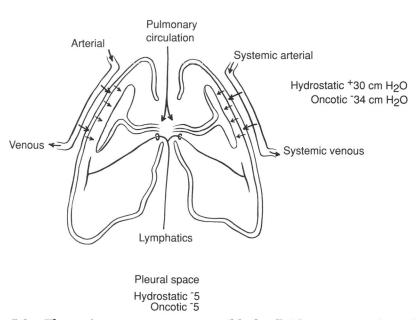

Pulmonary circulation ⁻hydrostatic ⁺11 cm H_2O
(to align)

Pulmonary
circulation

Arterial

Systemic arterial

Hydrostatic ⁺30 cm H_2O
Oncotic ⁻34 cm H_2O

Venous

Systemic venous

Lymphatics

Pleural space
Hydrostatic ⁻5
Oncotic ⁻5

Figure 5-2.   The various pressures responsible for fluid movement through the pleura.

circulation (see Chapter 7). Because it lines all five lobes and the lateral aspects of the mediastinum, it is much larger than the parietal pleura. Pulmonary capillary hydrostatic pressure is $+11$ cm H_2O; oncotic pressure is -34 cm H_2O. This difference results in a net pull of 23 cm H_2O of fluid out of the pleural space and into pulmonary circulation (Figure 5-2).

At any moment in time, there is an extremely small amount of fluid in the pleural space (<10 mL). The pH of the fluid is normally alkaline (pH 7.65). There is a substantial movement of fluid through this area, possibly 5–10 L per day. This fluid comes from the arterial end of the parietal pleura capillaries and is reabsorbed by the venous end of the visceral pleura capillaries. Excess fluid is removed by the pleural lymphatics.

The continuous tendency of the lung to pull away from the chest wall creates a negative pressure in the pleural space. Because of gravity and the weight of the lung (in an upright position) there is an additional pull in the apex of the lung (Figure 5-3). This results in more negative pressure being generated in the apex of the lung. The pressures are not just variable from the apex to the base of the lung, they are also variable during inspiration and expiration. As the chest wall and diaphragm pull out during inspiration, a greater negative pressure is generated throughout the potential pleural space. The difference accounts for approximately 0.25 cm H_2O/cm lung height. There-

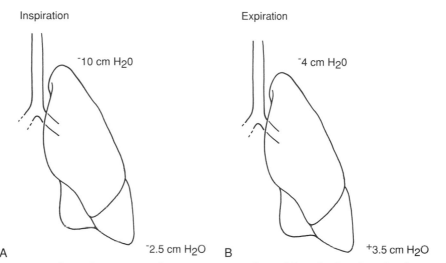

Inspiration

$^-$10 cm H_2O

Expiration

$^-$4 cm H_2O

A $^-$2.5 cm H_2O B $^+$3.5 cm H_2O

Figure 5-3. Pleural pressures in spontaneous breathing during inspiration and expiration.

fore, in the upright position, a lung height of 28 cm would result in a pressure difference of 7 cm H_2O, as shown in Figure 5-3. At the end of a deep inspiration, pleural apical pressures may be as low as -40 cm H_2O.

Pleural Fluid Testing

When fluid builds up in this region, lung space is occupied. Because the resulting loss of lung function can be devastating, effective treatment is imperative. In order for treatment to be effective, an accurate diagnosis is necessary. Aspiration and analysis of the accumulated fluid (pleural effusion) can be an important part of the diagnostic regimen (Figure 5-4).

Pleural effusions may be transudative or exudative. Transudate results from fluid entering the pleural space from the pulmonary capillary. This fluid has few blood cells and little protein. Exudate results when the pleural surfaces are diseased and the fluid contains a high protein content and cellular debris.

▼ ALVEOLAR GAS CONCENTRATIONS

Gas volume contained in the lung is essential to alveolar stability. The presence of a nonconsumable gas such as nitrogen is important in this regard. It provides a stable volume of gas to splint the gas exchange regions. O_2 is a consumable gas because it is removed from the lungs at a rate of approximately 250 mL/min. If continuous and adequate alveolar ventilation (V_A) is not sustained, gradual collapse and atelectasis will result.

Thoracentesis to aspirate pleural fluid

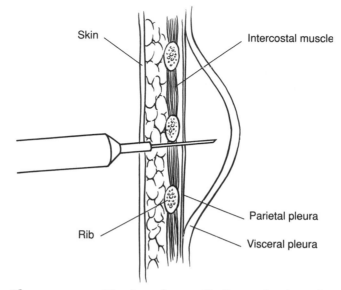

Figure 5-4.   The proper positioning of a needle for aspiration of accumulated fluid in the pleura.

The concentration of O_2 and CO_2 in an alveolus is dependent on a number of factors:

1. Ventilation per unit of time, breathing rate, and size of V_T (minute ventilation)
2. Distribution of ventilation
3. Concentration of inspired gases
4. Respiratory exchange ratio, removal of O_2, and input of CO_2 into the alveolus

Ventilation per Unit of Time

Alteration in respiratory rate (RR) or V_T can effect changes in ventilation per unit of time. If RR is increased, there is normally an increase in the amount of O_2 available and CO_2 removed. This would increase alveolar O_2 levels and decrease alveolar CO_2 levels. It will occur only if there is an increase in V_A.

Example #1

$$V_T = \text{Deadspace volume} + \text{Alveolar volume}$$

Normally,

$$V_T = 150 \text{ mL } (30\%) + 350 \text{ mL } (70\%)$$
$$= 500 \text{ mL}$$
$$RR = 15 \text{ breaths/min} \times 500 \text{ mL } V_T$$
$$= 7,500 \text{ mL minute ventilation}$$

Therefore, deadspace ventilation (V_D) is calculated as

$$V_D \text{ minute ventilation} = 15 \text{ breaths/min} \times 150 \text{ mL}$$
$$= 2,250 \text{ mL}$$

This is wasted work because it does not take part in gas exchange.

Alveolar Ventilation

To determine the amount of gas that actually takes part in gas exchange, perform the following calculations.

$$V_A = 15 \text{ breaths/min} \times 350 \text{ mL}$$
$$= 5,250 \text{ mL}$$

If the rate of ventilation is increased or decreased, there will be a direct change in V_A and therefore a change in alveolar gas concentration. This will result from a change in the quantity of CO_2 and O_2 exchanged.

The same minute volume with a different relationship between V_T and RR will yield different results. Remember, anatomical deadspace remains relatively constant from a practical point of view.

Example #2

Even when using the same minute ventilation of 7,500 mL, it is possible to have an increased V_T and a decreased RR.

$$RR = 10/\text{min}$$
$$V_T = 750 \text{ mL}$$
$$\text{Minute volume} = 10 \times 750$$
$$= 7,500 \text{ mL}$$
$$V_D = 10 \times 150$$
$$= 1,500 \text{ mL}$$
$$V_A = 10 \times 600$$
$$= 6,000 \text{ mL}$$

Notice that with the same minute ventilation we have increased V_A, affecting the amount of gas exchange occurring at an alveolar level. Remember, however, that an increase in V_T also can create an increase in O_2 consumption because of the increase in work required to further expand the lung (increased work because of compliance).

Distribution of Ventilation

Regional changes in resistance and compliance result in a variation in gas concentration from one alveolar exchange unit to another. Some areas will be well ventilated with appropriate perfusion and will have a corresponding concentration of gas. Others will be poorly ventilated or perfused, resulting in inadequate gas exchange and the resulting abnormal alveolar gas concentration.

Concentration of Inspired Gas

Alveolar gas concentration can be dramatically affected by the concentration of inspired gas. In most cases, the fractional inspired O_2 concentration (FIO_2) is expressed as a percentage. If FIO_2 increases above 21%, alveolar O_2 concentration is increased. If a patient inhales CO_2 as a result of rebreathing dead-space, alveolar concentrations of CO_2 also increase. Because nitrogen is not consumed by the body and is in equilibrium with the tissues, it can act as a splint within the alveolus. High O_2 concentrations can wash out or remove nitrogen and tend to contribute to alveolar instability, promoting an effect known as **diffusion atelectasis**. In a diseased lung, high O_2 concentrations can turn a **shunt effect** (partial ventilation) into a **true shunt** (no ventilation), a concept described later in this text (see Chapter 8).

Respiratory Exchange Ratio, the Removal of Oxygen, and the Input of Carbon Dioxide

These factors also affect the alveolar gas concentrations. It must be remembered that O_2 is constantly being removed from the alveoli and replaced by CO_2 as it diffuses out of the blood. The result is a lower than ambient O_2 concentration and higher than ambient CO_2 concentration.

When the exchange ratio is <1, the net gas volume is in deficit. In other words, more O_2 is being removed than CO_2 replaced. This creates a potential for alveolar collapse (atelectasis). Without continuous replacement of net gas volume, an effect known as **stasis atelectasis** results.

Calculating Alveolar Gas Concentration of Oxygen

One can determine the alveolar gas concentration of O_2 by plugging the appropriate values into the following gas alveolar equation:

$$PAO_2 = (P_B - 47) FIO_2 - PaCO_2 [(FIO_2 + 1 - FIO_2)/R]$$

The resultant value is calculated in mmHg pressure. The variables necessary for computing this value are as follows:

PAO_2 = the partial pressure of O_2 in the alveolus

P_B = barometric pressure − 47 mmHg; 47 is the water vapor pressure 100% saturated at 37°C because this is the vapor pressure in alveolar gas

FIO_2 = fractional inspired O_2 concentration expressed as a decimal. This considers the partial pressure of dry gases and accounts for the need to subtract the water vapor pressure first.

$PaCO_2$ = partial pressure of CO_2 in arterial blood. This is used to equate alveolar CO_2 concentration ($PACO_2$).

R = respiratory exchange ratio, which is the relationship between O_2 consumed and CO_2 produced in milliliters per minute:

$$R = CO_2 \text{ produced}/O_2 \text{ consumed}$$
$$= 200 \text{ (mL/min)}/250 \text{ (mL/min)}$$
$$= 0.8$$

Example #3

$$
\begin{array}{cc}
\text{(Part 1)} & \text{(Part 2)} \\
PAO_2 = (760 - 47)\, 0.21 & - 40\, [\{0.21 + (1 - 0.21)\}/0.8] \\
= 150 \text{ mmHg} & - 48 \\
= 102 \text{ mmHg}
\end{array}
$$

Part 1

The first part of the equation represents the partial pressure of O_2. It is determined by first calculating the total gas pressure dry. This is calculated by taking the barometric pressure (760 mmHg in this case) and subtracting the water vapor pressure of alveolar gas 100% saturated at 37°C (47 mmHg). The partial pressure of O_2 is then obtained by multiplying the total gas pressure dry by the fraction of this pressure that exists as O_2, in this case it is 0.21, or 21%.

Part 2

This part of the equation reflects the amount of O_2 being removed from the alveolar O_2 pressure. O_2 is being removed from the alveoli approximately 20% faster than CO_2 is being replaced. This constant removal of gas from the alveolar region (constant depletion of FRC) partially explains the need for a sigh (Figure 5-5).

Sigh

A deep breath close to total lung capacity is taken 14–18 times per hour depending on environmental, emotional, and individual differences. Failure to sigh over a period of time may result in stasis atelectasis, a common problem in patients with restricted chest movement (i.e., after abdominal or thoracic surgery). The importance of a sigh in lung clearance and stability should not be overlooked.

The sigh is a normal physiological activity that is very difficult, if not impossible, to reproduce with a mechanical ventilator. The respiratory therapist must therefore rely on deep breathing, coughing exercises, and early patient mobility to achieve the therapeutic effect. Because the sigh is a physical maneuver that pulls on the lung from the outside, it creates a lateral traction on the lung, which reduces both vascular and airway resistance.

▼ SURFACTANT

As discussed earlier, the lungs have a continual tendency to collapse because the volume of O_2 removed from the alveolar space is not totally replaced by CO_2. There are two other reasons for this:

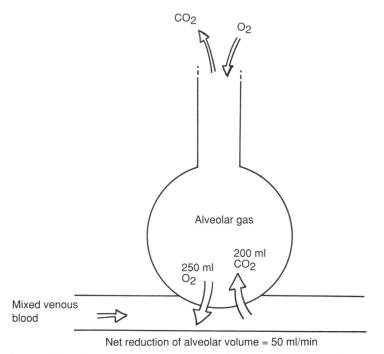

Figure 5-5.   The normal ongoing volume deficit in the lung.

1. Elastic recoil of the lungs
2. Surface tension of the alleged fluid lining in the alveoli

A fluid lining in the lung would cause the alveoli to collapse because of the intermolecular attraction between the surface molecules of the alveolar fluid. Surfactant, a lipoprotein secreted by type II alveolar cells, acts to reduce the surface-attractive forces between molecules (see Chapter 6). This makes lung expansion much easier, considerably reducing the work of breathing. Surfactant also appears to play a role in preventing the accumulation of fluid in the alveoli (pulmonary edema). Some believe it works as a water-proofing agent by combining with the cell membranes of alveolar type I and type II cells at a molecular level, thus producing a hydrophobic surface. The role of surfactant in the lungs remains controversial in terms of its mode of action. However, its importance in lung stability is not in question.

Two considerably different models can be used to describe the role of surfactant in the lungs when trying to explain the various phenomena encountered in clinical practice: the wet lung model and the dry lung model. The wet lung model, which describes surfactant in a liquid phase, is by far the more popular of the two.

Wet Lung Model

This model assumes that an enormous air–water interface lines the alveoli. The surface tension resulting from this interface produces forces that tend to reduce the overall area. The pressure tending to cause collapse of the lung depends on

1. the surface tension of the liquid in dynes per centimeter
2. the radius of the bubble in centimeters

This is expressed in the Laplace equation:

Pressure with the bubble (P)

$$= [2 \times \text{surface tension of the liquid}] / \text{radius of the bubble (R)}$$

$$P = [2T \, (\text{dynes/cm})] / R \, (\text{cm})$$

$$P = \text{dynes/cm}^2$$

The normal pressure within this bubble is approximately 4 cm H_2O. This low pressure is a result of the presence of surfactant. If pure water were lining the alveoli, the pressure would be approximately 15 cm H_2O. This would make lung volume maintenance extremely difficult and result in a significant increase in the work of breathing.

If the Laplace equation is used for our lung model, we will expect pressure to increase and smaller alveoli to empty into larger alveoli as one region of the lung becomes smaller than another. These lung regions become progressively smaller as pressures, increasing in smaller alveoli, cause collapse. This would eventually result in one larger alveolar unit. Progressively, this larger region would begin to collapse. In fact, the elastic recoil of smaller alveoli is less than that of the larger alveoli. This results from the presence of surfactant, which becomes more concentrated as the alveolar surfaces decrease in size.

Fluid movement into the lung from the capillary bed (pulmonary transudation) affects surfactant activity. The combination of surface tension and pulmonary capillary pressures favors the movement of fluid into the alveoli. These pressures are counteracted by the osmotic pressure of plasma proteins pulling fluid back into the capillary bed. If the influence of surfactant were sufficiently reduced, surface tension in the alveoli would increase, thus favoring fluid movement into the alveolus. The existence of fluid in the alveolus further reduces the effectiveness of surfactant, causing further aggravation of the problem. Obviously, excess fluid within alveolar air spaces would interfere with gas exchange. Surfactant function or presence can be affected by

1. pulmonary edema
2. immature lungs at birth (idiopathic respiratory distress syndrome)
3. extracorporeal perfusion, after open-heart surgery

Dry Lung Model

This alternative to the wet lung model was described by Hill in 1983.[*] Although it has never gained widespread acceptance, this model provides an extremely

---

[*]Hill BA, et al. Role of surfactant in the lungs and other organs. *Crit Care Med* 1983;11:12.

attractive and viable alternative to the wet lung model, mainly because it answers several questions not directly addressed by the wet lung model. According to the dry lung model, surfactant can be directly attached to solid surfaces if the charges are favorable.

In this case, we do not have a liquid lining with which to contend. Surfactant orients itself to attach directly to the alveolar epithelial lining. The attachment results in a dry hydrophobic surface, ideal for gas diffusion (without a liquid lining) and possessing none of the surface tension resulting from a liquid lining. This dry alveolar surface resists water (hydrophobic): water beads up (as it would in a Teflon frying pan) and rolls off into the corners, where it is absorbed into the *interstitium*, the small spaces between cells. Without the liquid lining, alveolar stability and gas diffusion would be enhanced.

▼ PARENCHYMAL ELASTICITY

Hooke's law describes elastic behavior in terms of the tension developed when an elastic structure is stretched. It states that the tension developed is proportional to the amount of deformation. In the lung, parenchymal yellow elastin fibers provide this physical elastic structure, tending to cause collapse of alveolar structures.

▼ CONCLUSION

The pleura, alveolar gas concentration, surfactant, and parenchymal elasticity are all important factors in maintaining an adequate FRC. (See Clinical Applications Box 5-1 for a discussion of maintaining oxygenation in the face of reduced lung volume.) It should be recognized that for gas exchange to be adequate, a continuous volume of gas must interface with blood in the lungs. The following two chapters address this relationship by exploring, respectively, pulmonary gas exhange and pulmonary circulation.

Clinical Applications Box 5-1   Continuous Positive Airway Pressure

When disease significantly affects lung volumes, oxygenation becomes a clinical problem. The most common reason for this is a reduction in compliance. It results in a decreased surface area for gas exchange with a direct affect on the patient's ability to take in O_2. Applying a positive pressure inside the lung can push it out and compensate for the increased tendency of the lung to collapse. This restoration of FRC can reestablish an acceptable level of oxygenation.

The positive pressure used in this case must be continuous if the FRC is to be constantly maintained. Today, many devices are available with the ability to provide this continuous positive airway pressure.

❖ Review Questions

1. Systemic capillary hydrostatic pressure is approximately
   a. 4 cm H_2O.
   b. 10 cm H_2O.
   c. 14 cm H_2O.
   d. 30 cm H_2O.
   e. 34 cm H_2O.
2. Pulmonary capillary hydrostatic pressure is approximately
   a. 4 cm H_2O.
   b. 11 cm H_2O.
   c. 23 cm H_2O.
   d. 30 cm H_2O.
   e. 34 cm H_2O.
3. The pH of pleural fluid is normally
   a. 7.35.
   b. 7.40.
   c. 7.45.
   d. 7.55.
   e. 7.65.
4. The greater negative pressure generated from the base to the apex of the lung is approximately _____ cm H_2O/cm lung height.
   a. 0.25
   b. 0.75
   c. 6.3
   d. 7
   e. 28
5. A transudative pleural effusion contains
   i. few blood cells.
   ii. cellular debris.
   iii. little protein.
   iv. red blood cells.
   v. bacteria.

   a. i, ii
   b. i, iii
   c. ii, iii, iv
   d. iii, iv, v
   e. ii, iv, v
6. Calculate the PAO_2 given the following information:
   $$P_B = 760 \text{ mmHg}$$
   $$FIO_2 = 0.21$$
   $$PaCO_2 = 40 \text{ mmHg}$$
   $$R = 0.8$$
   a. 102
   b. 150

    c. 149

    d. 197

    e. 215

7. Surfactant is

    i. a lipoprotein.

    ii. secreted by type II Λ secretory cells.

    iii. concentrated in the terminal bronchial.

    iv. secreted by type II alveolar cells.

    v. responsible for reducing surface tension.

    a. i, ii, iii

    b. iii, iv, v

    c. i, iv, v

    d. i, ii, v

    e. ii, iii, iv

6

▼

PULMONARY GAS EXCHANGE

OBJECTIVES

1. Describe the blood/gas interface in the lung.

2. List the barriers to gas diffusion from the alveoli into the blood and back to the alveoli.

3. Characterize the alveolar–capillary membrane.

4. Discuss the pressure gradient within the lung in terms of alveolar ventilation, capillary blood flow, and chemical reactions.

5. Define the relationship between diffusion and the physical characteristics of a gas.

Matthews LR: CARDIOPULMONARY ANATOMY AND PHYSIOLOGY. © 1996 Lippincott–Raven Publishers.

6. Explain diffusion capacity.
7. Identify the factors affecting pulmonary diffusion capacity.
8. Define diffusion block.
9. Describe spontaneous gas absorption.

Once the alveoli have been adequately ventilated, the exchange of carbon dioxide (CO_2) and oxygen (O_2) across the alveolar membrane becomes possible. The combination of the extremely large interface between blood and alveolar gas (approximately 75–100 m^2) and the thinness of the alveolar membrane separating blood from gas (approximately 0.5–1.0 μm) are the two primary factors responsible for promoting gas exchange. This relationship between gas and blood in the lung is most commonly referred to as the ventilation/perfusion relationship (V/Q) and will be discussed in Chapter 8, after we have addressed pulmonary gas exchange and pulmonary circulation.

Molecules of O_2 and CO_2 pass each other as they move across the pressure gradient during gas exchange. A freeze frame of this diffusion process would show little more than 2 L of functional residual capacity (FRC) interfacing with approximately 70–100 mL of blood. Remember that very little of the FRC (the amount of air left in the lung after normal expiration) is in direct contact with the alveolar–capillary (A/C) interface. It is amazing to think that such a small volume of gas and blood are spread out over such a vast area. However, it does make the delicate nature of this system very apparent. Anything that disrupts either blood or air flow will have a dramatic effect on gas exchange.

The normal aerobic metabolic process in the body uses O_2, which must make its way into the cell, and produces CO_2, which must make its way out of the cell. The same barriers to exchange are present for each of these gases even though they move in opposite directions: air passes into the cells in O_2 form and cells, in turn, release CO_2 into the air (Table 6-1). This chapter will deal with diffusion of gas from the alveolus into the blood and the various factors affecting this process.

▼ THE ALVEOLAR–CAPILLARY MEMBRANE

Alveolar–Capillary Membrane Anatomy

The *alveolar–capillary (A/C) membrane* is a fusion of the capillary wall and the alveolar wall against a common basement membrane. It consists of *capillary*

TABLE 6-1 Barriers to Diffusion		
CO_2	Alveolar capillary membrane Blood plasma Red blood cell Capillary, interstitium, and cell membrane Cytoplasm and the mitochondria	O_2

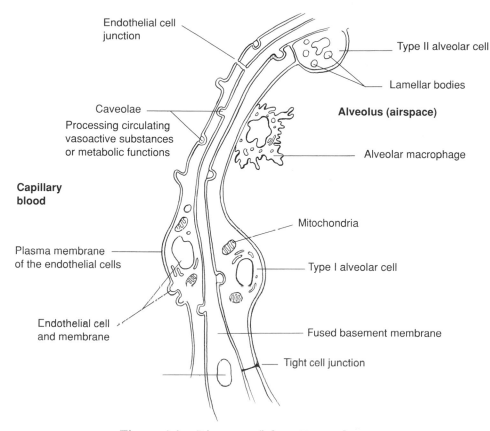

Figure 6-1. Diagram of the A/C membrane.

endothelial cells, a basement membrane, and type I (squamous pneumocytes) and type II (granular pneumocytes) alveolar cells (Figure 6-1). The capillary endothelium is a continuous bricklike layer of cells supported by the underlying basement membrane. The basement membrane is important because it provides structural support for the capillary bed and the alveolar surface.

Type I cells are flat and thin, making up the vast majority of the gas exchange area (approximately 95%). Type II cells are thick, highly active cells responsible for the production of surfactant, which is stored in lamellar bodies

---

Preview Box 6.1 Pulmonary Capillary Network

This massive network of blood vessels provides the interface between the lungs and the circulatory system. The venous side of this capillary network is filled with oxygenated blood returning from the lungs. See Chapter 7.

inside the cell. Free-floating cells inside the alveolus engulf and ingest material foreign to the alveolar surface. These *alveolar macrophages*, or type III cells, are important in protecting the lung from invasion (see Chapter 15).

The rate of diffusion of a gas across a membrane can be influenced by a number of membrane-associated factors, such as its thickness and the viscosity of the liquid through which the gas passes.

The Thickness of the Membrane

The thickness of the alveolar membrane varies throughout the lung but is usually 0.5–1.0 μm.

The thickness of the A/C membrane can be increased if fluid enters the interstitium. Fluid accumulation in the interstitium (interstitial edema) may be the result of

1. increased capillary hydrostatic pressure
2. obstructed lymphatic flow
3. reduced blood osmotic pressure
4. membrane trauma (type I and type II cells)

Interstitial edema can potentially impede adequate diffusion by increasing the distance over which the gases are spread. Certain other interstitial diseases, which include the occupational lung diseases and sarcoidosis, can result in fibrosis (scarring) in the aftermath of chronic or acute inflammation. The resulting reduction in lung volume plays a significant role in reducing diffusion, generally by reducing the surface area involved in gas exchange.

Liquid Viscosity

The diffusion rate is inversely related to the viscosity of the fluid through which the gas is diffusing. Because the viscosity of the alveolar liquid lining is relatively constant, it is not considered a variable under normal circumstances. However, liquid viscosity does become a factor in the interstitial diseases.

▼ SURFACE AREA

As mentioned at the beginning of this chapter, surface area of the respiratory system is normally 75–100 m². This large surface area is extremely important if adequate diffusion is to occur. Anything that can decrease surface area decreases diffusion capacity. Removing a lung or a part of the lung has this effect. Emphysema also results in a significant reduction in surface area as the alveolar walls deteriorate.

When the surface area is reduced so that it accommodates less than half the normal diffusion capacity, it has been reduced enough to have a significant impact on the patient, even at rest. The normal diffusion capacity for O_2 is approximately 31 mL O_2/min/mmHg pressure gradient. Carbon monoxide is used for diffusion tests because, in the presence of a normal amount of hemoglobin and normal ventilatory function, the status of the A/C membrane is the main limiting factor to carbon monoxide diffusion rate.

▼ PRESSURE GRADIENT

This gradient is formed by the difference in the partial pressure of O_2 (PO_2) and the partial pressure of CO_2 (PCO_2) between alveolar and capillary gas. Gas always moves from a high to a low pressure (Figure 6-2). Venous blood return-

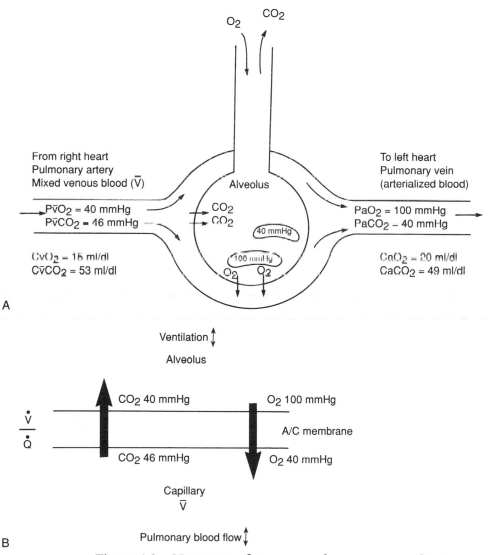

Figure 6-2. Movement of gas across the pressure gradient.

ing from the body is relatively low in O_2 pressure and high in CO_2 pressure, which creates the ideal condition under which CO_2 can efficiently exit the body.

The rate of gas exchange and the volume of gas exchanged is directly related to the gas pressure difference between alveolar and capillary gases. The greater the pressure difference, the larger the gas movement. Three primary factors contribute to maintaining this pressure gradient:

1. Alveolar ventilation
2. Pulmonary capillary blood flow
3. Chemical reactions

Alveolar Ventilation

Normal ventilation results in an arterial partial pressure of O_2 (PaO_2) of 80–100 mmHg and a normal partial pressure of CO_2 ($PaCO_2$) of 35–45 mmHg. During hyperventilation, alveolar gas concentration approaches the concentration of inspired air.

Extreme hyperventilation can result in a PaO_2 approaching 150 mmHg (ambient PO_2) and a $PaCO_2$ <10 mmHg, resulting in alkalosis. Extreme hypoventilation can have the opposite effect, resulting in a PaO_2 of <50 mmHg and a $PaCO_2$ well in excess of 50 mmHg.

In order to achieve adequate ventilation, it is essential that the ventilatory pattern match the body's metabolic demands. Although short-term hyper- or hypoventilation can be easily handled by the body and normal metabolic processes, long-term disturbances can be extremely troublesome or even devastating because of the resulting alkalosis (excessive alkalinity of body fluids) or acidosis (excessive acidity of body fluids). These metabolic disturbances are covered in Chapter 14.

Pulmonary Capillary Blood Flow

As venous blood enters the pulmonary capillary bed it has a PO_2 of approximately 40 mmHg and a PCO_2 of approximately 46 mmHg. As it moves through a ventilated alveolus, the PO_2 begins to increase and the PCO_2 decreases (Figure 6-3).

The diffusion rate is extremely high initially; it tapers off as the concentration gradient decreases. If the demand for O_2 uptake and CO_2 removal is increased (as in exercise), a greater pressure gradient is created and the diffusion rate increases as long as alveolar ventilation is increased correspondingly.

Chemical Reactions

The large volume of O_2 and CO_2 carried by the blood is dependent on the *erythrocyte* (red blood cell) and its content of hemoglobin molecules. Without hemoglobin, the blood would fill almost instantaneously as it contacted the

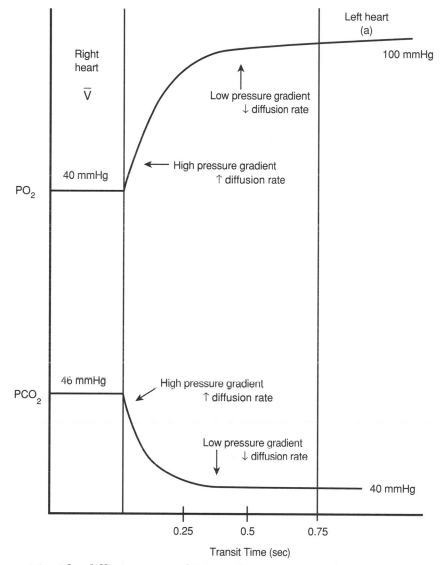

Figure 6-3.   The diffusion rates of PO$_2$ and PCO$_2$ in seconds as they move through an alveolus.

Preview Box 6-2   Red Blood Cells and Hemoglobin

Chapter 9 is devoted to the topic of gas transport via red blood cells (RBCs or erythrocytes), particularly hemoglobin's unique affinity for the gases exchanged during ventilation. Although the chapter is grounded in the normal physiology of gas transport, it dedicates a fair amount of time to the exploration of abnormalities in gas transport. See Chapter 9.

A/C membrane and would contain only 0.3 mL per 100 mL of blood. Hemoglobin, which acts as a reservoir, is filled with and emptied of gases as necessary.

Normally blood enters the pulmonary circulation approximately 75% full of O_2 and leaves 98–100% full of O_2. This process generally requires the addition of 5 mL of O_2 for every 100 mL of blood. Venous content is normally 15 mL per 100 mL and the arterial content is 20 mL per 100 mL of blood.

CO_2 also relies on erythrocytes as its principal means of transport. Without the red blood cells' and hemoglobin's unique affinity for these gases, our bodies could not carry sufficient quantities of CO_2 to satisfy our metabolic needs.

As CO_2 leaves the blood, it is continuously replenished by CO_2 leaving the red blood cell. This maintains an adequate pressure gradient across the A/C membrane. Venous blood entering the lung has a content of approximately 53 mL of CO_2 per 100 mL of blood and leaves with 49 mL of CO_2 per 100 mL of blood as it enters pulmonary veins on its way to the left side of the heart.

Carbonic anhydrase exists in the alveolar epithelium. This enzyme promotes the dissociation of CO_2 and H_2O into hydrogen (H^+) and bicarbonate (HCO_3^-). The resulting small pressure gradient is then maintained to facilitate diffusion of the large amount of CO_2 needed with such a small pressure gradient (5–6 mmHg).

▼ THE PHYSICAL CHARACTERISTICS OF THE GAS

Three things must be considered with respect to variability of diffusion from one gas to another:

1. Molecular weight of the gas
2. Gas solubility in body fluids
3. Gas temperature

Molecular Weight of the Gas

Larger gas molecules move through a membrane more slowly than do smaller ones. Graham's law states that the relative rates of diffusion for two gases are inversely proportional to the square roots of their molecular weights (see

Appendix 2). Based on Graham's law alone, O_2 has a molecular weight lower than that of CO_2.

Example #1

$CO_2/O_2 = 44/32 = 1.17$

According to this law, O_2 would be 1.17 times more diffusible than CO_2.

Gas Solubility (Solubility Coefficient)

For our purposes, solubility is measured in milliliters of gas dissolved in each 100 mL of blood per mmHg pressure at 37°C (mL/100 mL blood/mmHg/37°C).

The rate of diffusion across a biological membrane depends on its ability to dissolve into body fluids. Using this as a criterion, there is a major difference between O_2 and CO_2. The solubility coefficient of O_2 is 0.003 mL/100 mL blood/mmHg/37°C, whereas the solubility of CO_2 is 0.067 mL/100 mL blood/mmHg/37°C. CO_2 is approximately 20 times more soluble in plasma than O_2.

Henry's law describes the relationship between partial pressure and the solubility coefficient by defining the weight of a gas dissolved in a given volume of liquid (at a constant temperature) to be directly proportional to pressure (see Appendix 2). Mathematically speaking, this is expressed as follows:

Concentration = gas pressure × solubility of dissolved gas coefficient solubility

This difference in solubility between CO_2 and O_2 far outweighs the diffusion difference attributable to molecular weight. CO_2 diffuses much faster than O_2 across the A/C membrane. This factor is significant in clinical practice because it is the main reason O_2 levels are affected before CO_2 levels in the early phases of lung disease. Although solubility is extremely important in the diffusion of gas across the A/C membrane, little is actually carried in this dissolved form.

Example #2

Arterial blood carries approximately 20 mL of O_2 per 100 mL of blood. In solution,

Normal $PaO_2 = 100$ mmHg

Solubility coefficient of $O_2 = 0.003$ mL/100 mL/mmHg/37°C

Therefore,

$100 \times 0.003 = 0.3$ mL/100 mL of blood

If the total amount of O_2 carried is 20 mL/100 mL and only 0.3 mL is carried in solution, <2% is carried in solution. The rest is carried by hemoglobin (approximately 1.34 mL/g hemoglobin). It is the gas that is carried in solution that is essential to gas transfer in and out of the blood.

Gas Temperature

Increased body temperature results in an increase in diffusion rate. The normal lung temperature is 37°C and in healthy individuals will not change significantly. During exercise, skeletal muscle temperature can increase significantly enough to elevate the gas diffusion rate, thus promoting gas exchange. Increased temperature also promotes the release of O_2 by hemoglobin and increases O_2 consumption by the tissue.

▼ DIFFUSION

Facilitated Diffusion

Cytochrome P-450

This is a hemoprotein enzyme attached to the endoplasmic reticulum within the cells of the A/C membrane. It is thought to facilitate the diffusion of O_2 across the A/C membrane. It may be responsible for as much as 10–15% of the O_2 transported per unit time.

Myoglobin

Skeletal and cardiac muscles have relatively high concentrations of myoglobin within their cell cytoplasm. With a molecular weight one fourth that of hemoglobin, this heme protein attaches to and stores O_2 because of its high affinity for the O_2 molecule. It actually has a higher affinity for O_2 than does hemoglobin, which is unable to release O_2, except at low O_2 tensions. It is also important in the facilitated transport of O_2 into the muscle cells.

The myoglobin molecule has a structure similar to the subunits of the hemoglobin molecule (globin polypeptide chains). Increased temperature is the only factor known to diminish myoglobin's affinity for O_2.

Diffusion Capacity

Pulmonary diffusion capacity is a measurement of the volume of a specific gas that can be transferred per unit of time across the A/C membrane. It combines all of the diffusion concepts previously discussed.

The following statements can be made about the variability of diffusion capacity:

1. It is directly proportional to the pressure gradient across the membrane.
2. It is directly proportional to the solubility of the gas in the membrane.
3. It is inversely proportional to the membrane thickness.
4. It is inversely proportional to the molecular weight of the diffusing gas.

5. It is directly proportional to the reaction rate of O_2 with hemoglobin.
6. It is directly proportional to the volume of blood in the capillary bed.

Fick's law of diffusion describes the factors influencing gas flow through the A/C membrane (see Appendix 2) and is expressed as follows:

$$\dot{V} \text{ gas} = A \times D/T \times (P_1 - P_2)$$

where $\dot{V}$ = alveolar ventilation, A = cross-sectional area available for diffusion (direct relationship with diffusion), D = diffusion coefficient of the gas (also a direct relationship), T = thickness of the membrane (an indirect relationship), and $(P_1 - P_2)$ = pressure gradient across the membrane (a direct relationship with diffusion).

Factors Affecting Pulmonary Diffusion Capacity

Diffusion capacity is influenced by a number of factors, most notably body position and size, exercise, and the presence of disease.

Body Position

Diffusion capacity is increased by up to 20% when the patient is in a recumbent position. Gravity is primarily responsible for this because

1. when a patient lies down, blood supply in the lung is more evenly distributed across the lung fields (improved ventilation/perfusion matching [$\dot{V}/\dot{Q}$]).
2. pulmonary blood volume increases.

Body Size

An individual's body size (as determined by approximation to ideal body weight) relates directly to the size of his or her A/C membrane. Diffusion capacity is increased as the ventilation perfusion interface is increased. However, it should be noted that increasing body size by eating excessively will do nothing to increase the size of the lungs.

Exercise

Diffusion capacity increases as much as 35% during exercise. This results from a combination of the following factors:

1. Increased alveolar ventilation
2. Increased capillary blood volume
3. Improved blood distribution ($\dot{V}/\dot{Q}$ improved)
4. Increased hemoglobin concentration as a result of sympathetic discharge and fluid shifts in prolonged exercise

Disease

The A/C interface can be reduced by any of the following processes:

1. Destruction of alveolar and capillary tissue (emphysema) (Figure 6-4)

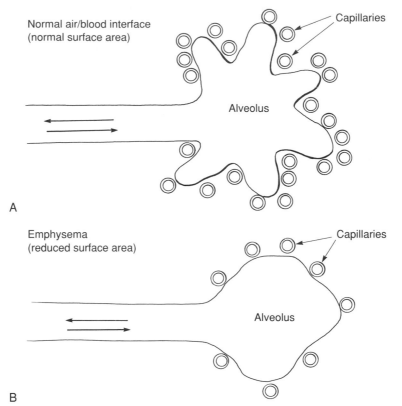

Figure 6-4.   Emphysema leads to a reduction of the surface area covered by the A/C interface.

2. Obstruction of an airway (mucus plug) or consolidation of a gas exchange region (pneumonia) inhibiting gas flow (Figure 6-5a)
3. Capillary blood flow obstruction (pulmonary embolism) (Figure 6-5b)
4. Mismatch of ventilation and perfusion results when the majority of blood flow is not entering the same regions as the majority of gas flow ($\dot{V}/\dot{Q}$ mismatch). This situation generally results from a combination of (1) and (2).

Diffusion Block

Increased thickness of the A/C membrane also decreases diffusion capacity, although it is much less significant than the $\dot{V}/\dot{Q}$ relationship. This condition has been referred to as a diffusion block. It may be caused by

1. alveolar fibrosis (scarring as a result of tissue damage). It is more likely that the diffusion capacity is decreased because of the reduced compliance and resulting reduction in ventilation.

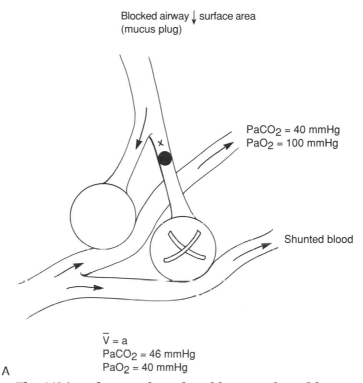

Blocked airway ↓ surface area
(mucus plug)

$PaCO_2$ = 40 mmHg
PaO_2 = 100 mmHg

Shunted blood

$\overline{V}$ = a
$PaCO_2$ = 46 mmHg
PaO_2 = 40 mmHg

A

Figure 6-5.   The A/C interface can be reduced by a number of factors, among them (a) blocking of an airway with a mucus plug and (b) the obstruction of capillary blood flow such as occurs during a pulmonary embolism.

2. alveolar interstitial edema (swelling of the A/C membrane). The accumulation of fluid in the area between the vasculature and the alveoli is most commonly a result of pulmonary hypertension and lymphatic overload.

We have now recognized that diffusion blocks are much less significant than the $\dot{V}/\dot{Q}$ mismatch usually present at the same time (see Chapter 8). Pulmonary edema, silicosis, and sarcoidosis are examples of diseases that can disrupt the A/C membrane. Although they can reduce the diffusibility of O_2 and CO_2, much more significant is their ability to disrupt the ventilation and perfusion matchup, thereby effectively reducing surface area for diffusion.

▼ SPONTANEOUS GAS ABSORPTION

A gas bubble, or pocket, in the body gradually decreases in size until it disappears, and if its walls are rigid, it will develop a negative pressure. This can occur with a spontaneous pneumothorax (introduction of air into the lungs) or block-

Blocked capillary blood flow
(pulmonary embolism)

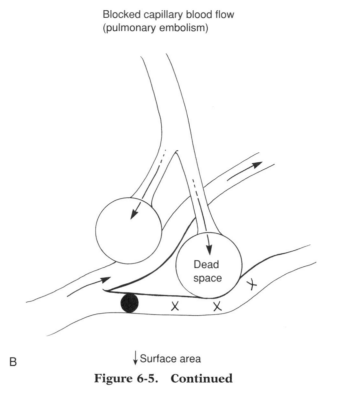

B   ↓Surface area

Figure 6-5.   Continued

age of an airway. In both cases, there is a closed pocket of gas, and equilibration between concentration of gases between the space and surrounding tissues occurs. There is a general deficit of gas pressure in the body (i.e., approximately 60 mmHg O_2 pressure is removed from the blood and replaced with 5 mmHg CO_2 pressure). Also, gas pockets generally have high O_2 concentration and low CO_2 concentration, further contributing to gas diffusion out of the area.

Remember that even in a healthy lung, a disparity in volume removed (O_2) versus volume added (CO_2) results in constant deflation of the lung. A normal exchange ratio between CO_2 and O_2 is approximately 0.8, meaning that for every 5 mL of O_2 removed from the lung, only 4 mL of CO_2 is replaced. This is partially responsible for the constant need for sighs to keep lung volume (FRC) up (see Chapter 5). If we breathe at a constant volume for long enough, alveolar collapse begins to occur (**stasis atelectasis**). The smaller the tidal volume, the more pronounced the effect (atelectasis occurs quickly). As this process develops, the area in which effective gas exchange can take place is gradually reduced.

▼ CONCLUSION

Diffusion of O_2 from the alveoli into the blood and diffusion of CO_2 from the blood into the alveoli is essential for life. The three most important factors to consider in this process are:

1. alveolar ventilation ($\dot{V}$)
2. pulmonary perfusion ($\dot{Q}$)
3. matching of the above two factors ($\dot{V}/\dot{Q}$ matching)

Ventilation and perfusion must match up directly for gas diffusion to occur. This ideal is reflective of an exact match between alveolar ventilation and the blood supply coming from the right heart. Because ventilation is affected by pressures in the pleurae related to gravitation, the upper portions of the lung receive relatively larger amounts of gas. The opposite is true with the blood supply: gravity causes blood to be more dominant in the lower portions of the lung.

If ventilation or perfusion is reduced in the lung, diffusion capacity is decreased. If the matching of ventilation and perfusion is offset, diffusion capacity is decreased. Any disease that results in disruption of either ventilation or pulmonary blood flow has a detrimental effect on gas diffusion. The next chapter will describe these variations in ventilation/perfusion.

❖ Review Questions

1. The surface area of the blood–gas interface in the lung is approximately (m^2)
   a. 25–50.
   b. 50–75.
   c. 75–100.
   d. 100–125.
   e. 125–150.
2. The A/C membrane is approximately (μm)
   a. 0.5–1.0.
   b. 1.0–2.0.
   c. 2.0–3.0.
   d. 3.0–4.0
   e. 5.0–6.0.
3. The volume of blood interfacing with gas in the lung is approximately (mL)
   a. 30–50.
   b. 50–70.
   c. 70–100.
   d. 100–200.
   e. 400–500.
4. Fluid accumulation in the alveolar interstitium may be a result of
   i. increased capillary hydrostatic pressure.
   ii. obstructed lymphatic flow.
   iii. reduced blood osmotic pressure.
   iv. membrane trauma.
   v. membrane fibrosing.

   a. i, ii, iii
   b. ii, iii, iv
   c. iii, iv, v
   d. i, iii, v
   e. All of the above

5. The normal diffusion capacity of the lung is approximately (in mL/ O_2/min/mmHg pressure gradient)
   a. 20.
   b. 30.
   c. 40.
   d. 50.
   e. 60.

6. The three primary factors that contribute to maintenance of the alveolar/blood gas pressure gradient are
   i.   alveolar ventilation.
   ii. membrane thickness.
   iii. pulmonary capillary blood flow.
   iv. alveolar deadspace.
   v.   chemical reactions.
   a. ii, iii, iv
   b. iii, iv, v
   c. i, iii, v
   d. ii, iii, v
   e. All of the above

7. Carbon dioxide is approximately _____ times more soluble than oxygen in plasma.
   a. 10
   b. 20
   c. 30
   d. 120
   e. 210

8. Cytochrome P-450 is
   i.   a hemoprotein.
   ii. attached to the endoplasmic reticulum within the A/C membrane.
   iii. thought to facilitate O_2 diffusion.
   iv. responsible for as much as 10–15% of O_2 transport across the A/C membrane
   v.   attached to hemoglobin.
   a. i, ii, iii
   b. ii, iii, iv
   c. iii, iv, v
   d. i, ii, iii, iv
   e. All of the above

9. Myoglobin
   i.   is in relatively high concentration in skeletal and cardiac muscle.
   ii. has a molecular weight four times that of hemoglobin.

    iii. stores oxygen.

    iv. decreases its attractive forces for O_2 in lower than normal temperature.

    v. has a higher affinity for oxygen than hemoglobin.

    a. i, ii, iii

    b. ii, iii, iv

    c. iii, iv, v

    d. i, iii, v

    e. All of the above

10. Diffusion capacity is

    i. inversely proportional to the pressure gradient.

    ii. inversely proportional to the solubility of the gas.

    iii. directly proportional to membrane thickness.

    iv. directly proportional to the molecular weight of the gas.

    v. directly proportional to blood volume in the capillary bed.

    a. v only

    b. i, ii, iii

    c. ii, iii, iv

    d. iii, iv, v

    e. All of the above

11. Diffusion capacity is influenced by

    i. cardiac output.

    ii. body position.

    iii. body size.

    iv. exercise.

    v. alveolar consolidation.

    a. i, ii, iii

    b. iii, iv, v

    c. i, iii, v

    d. i, ii, iii, iv

    e. All of the above

12. Emphysema results in

    a. decreased diffusion capacity.

    b. decreased capillary shunting.

    c. decreased alveolar deadspace.

    d. increased diffusion coefficient.

    e. reduced pulmonary vascular resistance.

13. Alveolar interstitial edema is most commonly associated with

    a. lymphatic insufficiency.

    b. alveolar fibrosis.

    c. reduced lung compliance.

    d. alveolar hyperventilation.

    e. pulmonary hypertension.

7

PULMONARY CIRCULATION

OBJECTIVES

1. Review the anatomy of the pulmonary circulation.

2. Discuss the function of the right side of the heart.

3. Describe the pulmonary vessels, bronchial vessels, and
   pulmonary lymphatics.

Matthews LR: CARDIOPULMONARY ANATOMY AND PHYSIOLOGY. © 1996 Lippincott–Raven Publishers.

4. Examine pulmonary interstitial fluid dynamics.

5. Define pulmonary edema and list the common causes of it.

6. Discuss the safety factor with respect to pulmonary edema.

7. State and describe the pressures associated with pulmonary circulation.

8. Explore the factors associated with pulmonary vascular smooth muscle tone.

9. Analyze the concept of pulmonary vascular compliance.

10. List and describe the factors affecting pulmonary blood volume.

11. Describe the pressures surrounding the pulmonary vasculature.

12. Explain the usefulness of monitoring pulmonary pressures.

13. Define wedge pressure.

14. List and describe the factors affecting blood distribution in the lung.

15. Describe the effect pulmonary vascular resistance has on blood flow through the pulmonary vessels.

16. List and characterize the most common pathologies associated with pulmonary vasculature.

17. Explain the metabolic functions of the lung.

Blood flow must come in direct contact with a ventilated alveolus if equilibration of oxygen (O_2) and carbon dioxide (CO_2) is to occur. Pulmonary circulation is routed through four major components to ensure that this state is achieved: the right side of the heart, pulmonary vessels, bronchial vessels, and lymphatics. All components of this system must be functioning effectively for sufficient quantities of O_2 and CO_2 to exchange places. Cardiac function, patent pulmonary vessels, blood pressure, fluid balance, and a healthy alveolar/capillary (A/C) membrane are all important considerations when investigating gas exchange abnormalities. This chapter describes the role of pulmonary circulation in the lung and the various factors affecting its efficiency.

▼ ANATOMY OF PULMONARY CIRCULATION

The Right Side of the Heart

The left ventricle contracts with such force that it protrudes into the right ventricle, assuming a crescent shape, as shown in Figure 7-1. The right ventricular muscle, because it is approximately one-third the thickness of its left coun-

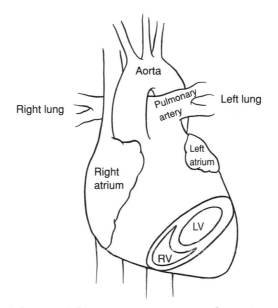

Figure 7-1. The right ventricle assumes a crescent shape to accommodate the forceful contraction of the left ventricle.

terpart, can yield to accommodate this contraction. This is primarily a result of the pressure difference in the two systems. The systolic (contractile) pressure created by the right side of the heart averages 25 mmHg, whereas the systolic pressure created by the left side of the heart averages 120 mmHg. The blood output is directly related to returning venous blood volume (see Chapter 10 for a description of this phenomenon.)

Pulmonary Vessels

The *pulmonary artery* leaves the right ventricle and splits into the right and left branches, each of which supplies blood to its respective lung. The wall of each pulmonary artery is about 30% the size of the aorta. The way in which these blood vessels branch mirrors the branching of the airways, all the way down to the terminal bronchioles (Figure 7-2), where they break into a massive network called the *pulmonary capillary bed*. The venous side of this capillary network is actually filled with oxygenated blood, which returns from the lung to form four large veins that drain into the left atrium.

The pulmonary arteries and *arterioles* have relatively large diameters and thin walls. These anatomical characteristics allow for a high compliance. The stroke volume output (volume output per beat) of the right ventricle is approximately 70 mL, and the compliance of the pulmonary vasculature is approximately 2 mL/mmHg. This means that with a normal systolic pulmonary pressure of 25 mmHg, 50 mL of the 70-mL cardiac output per beat can be

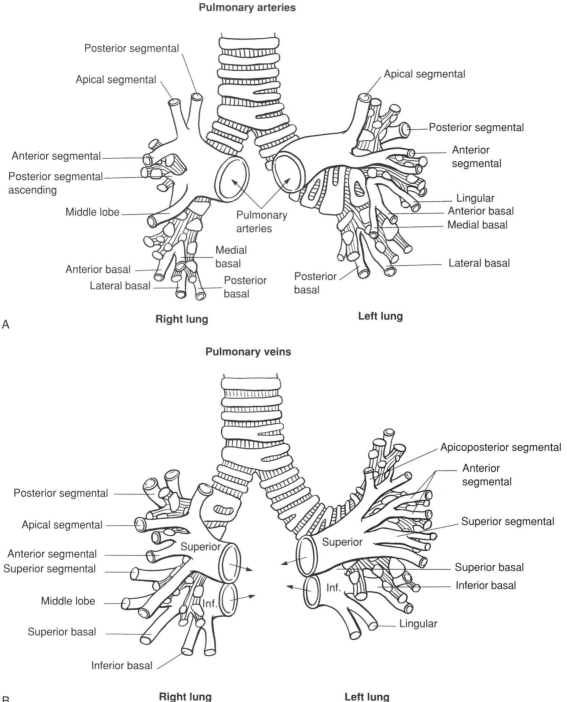

Pulmonary arteries

Posterior segmental

Apical segmental

Apical segmental

Posterior segmental

Anterior segmental

Anterior segmental

Posterior segmental ascending

Lingular

Middle lobe

Anterior basal

Pulmonary arteries

Medial basal

Medial basal

Lateral basal

Anterior basal

Lateral basal

Posterior basal

Posterior basal

Right lung

Left lung

A

Pulmonary veins

Apicoposterior segmental

Posterior segmental

Anterior segmental

Apical segmental

Superior segmental

Anterior segmental

Superior segmental

Superior

Superior

Superior basal

Middle lobe

Inf.

Inferior basal

Inf.

Superior basal

Lingular

Inferior basal

B

Right lung

Left lung

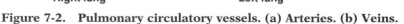

Figure 7-2.   Pulmonary circulatory vessels. (a) Arteries. (b) Veins.

accommodated by the vessels. This aids in keeping the system pressure relatively low.

Bronchial Vessels

Approximately 1–2% of the cardiac output supplies O_2 and nutrition for the lung-supporting tissues (i.e., connective tissue, the lung septa, and the large and small bronchi). The unusual thing about this blood supply is that once it passes through the tissues, it empties back into the pulmonary veins (and not central venous circulation) and enters the left side of the heart, producing an anatomic shunt, mixing venous or oxygenated blood with arterial blood. This also contributes to a slightly larger output from the left ventricle. The alveoli themselves are supplied with nutrients and cellular circulatory support by the pulmonary vessels.

Lymphatics

Lymphatic vessels arise from the tissue surrounding the vascular and bronchial spaces, run into the hilum of the lung, and then primarily empty into the right lymphatic duct. Lymphatic flow is approximately 5–6 mL/hr/100 g of lung tissue but, if necessary, it can increase 20-fold. This system is an alternate route by which fluids and particulate matter can enter the bloodstream. Because protein and large particles cannot be removed from the tissue spaces by normal absorption, it is left to the lymphatics to provide this function.

There are more lymphatic vessels in the lung per unit of tissue than in any other organ in the body. This may be a result of the extensive pulmonary interface with the environment and the corresponding need to remove particulate matter (see Chapters 12 and 15 for discussions of different aspects of the lymphatics).

Lymph Flow Out of the Lungs

Lymphatic fluid movement out of the lungs is controlled by the following three mechanisms: the lymphatic valves, the contraction of smooth muscle, and vessel compression.

Lymphatic Valves

These valves exist in all lymph channels. They are essential one-way check valves that appear every few millimeters along the vessels. Their placement ensures that fluid moves in one direction, out of the lung.

Smooth Muscle

The smooth muscle surrounding the lymph vessels can contract rhythmically in a peristaltic fashion, creating a wave of pressure that moves fluid. This process is aided considerably by the one-way check valves.

Vessel Compression

External forces acting to compress lymphatic vessels can have the same impact on flow as smooth muscle contraction. Changes in vascular and pulmonary pressure may result in this enhanced lymphatic flow.

The rate of lymph flow out of the lung and into the venous circulation can be increased by any of the following:

1. Increased capillary pressure
2. Decreased plasma osmotic pressure
3. Increased interstitial osmotic pressure
4. Increased pulmonary capillary permeability

Each of the above factors can cause pulmonary edema and disrupting gas exhange.

In summary, anything that increases interstitial fluid pressure or lymphatic pump activity will increase lymph flow out of the lungs.

▼ INTERSTITIAL FLUID DYNAMICS

The delicate nature of the pulmonary/alveolar–capillary (A/C) interface makes an understanding of fluid dynamics in the lung particularly important. Swelling of the A/C membrane and movement of fluid into the alveolar space can result in a major disruption of both alveolar gas distribution and capillary blood supply. Table 7-1 provides a useful series of comparisons between pulmonary and fluid systemic dynamics.

Fluid Balance Throughout the Alveolar–Capillary Membrane

Pressures that tend to move fluid out of the interstitial space are positive, and those responsible for movement of fluid into the interstitial space are negative (Figure 7-3).

The forces influencing the lung are both external, which tend to move fluid out of the pulmonary capillary bed, and internal, which tend to pull fluid into the pulmonary capillary bed. (Remember, fluid will move from an area of higher pressure to an area of lower pressure.) The following summary of external and internal forces illustrates the factors that have a role in interstitial fluid dynamics.

Total outward forces (pulmonary capillaries) = 30 mmHg

TABLE 7-1   Comparison of Pulmonary and Systemic Fluid Dynamics

1. Pulmonary capillary pressure averages 8 mmHg. Sytsemic capillary pressure averages 17 mmHg.
2. The pulmonary capillaries are relatively leaky to protein molecules in comparison with systemic capillaries.
3. The continuous pumping action in the lungs (thoracic pump) creates a very high rate of lymph flow (reduced during positive pressure mechanical ventilation).
4. The interstitial spaces in the gas exchange units of the lung are extremely narrow in comparison with those in other regions in the body.
5. The A/C membrane is between 0.5–1.0 μm thick, making it extremely susceptible to rupture.

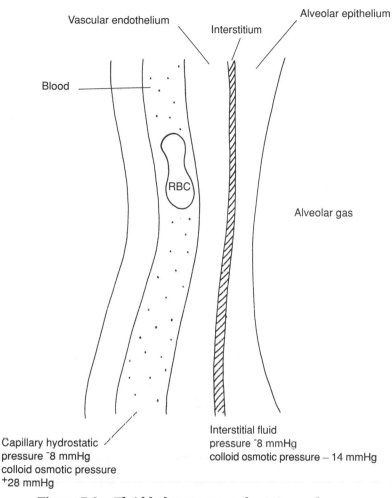

Figure 7-3.   **Fluid balance across the A/C membrane.**

1. Capillary hydrostatic pressures = 8 mmHg
2. Negative interstitial fluid pressures[*] = 8 mmHg
3. Interstitial fluid colloid osmotic = 14 mmHg pressures

Total inward forces (pulmonary capillaries) = 38 mmHg. (Inward force is completely dependent on plasma colloid osmotic pressure.)

1. Forces pushing out total 30 mmHg
2. Forces pushing in total 28 mmHg

[*]Negative interstitial fluid pressure is a poorly understood phenomenon. A negative interstitial pressure is one that has been measured and cannot be explained by simply looking at osmotic and hydrostatic pressure differences.

This results in a pressure excess of 2 mmHg, which pushes fluid into the interstitium. This region must be kept dry, and under normal circumstances this is accomplished effectively by the lymphatics.

Pulmonary Edema

Anything that disrupts the pressure balance of fluid movement between the capillary bed and the interstitium may result in a buildup of fluid (**edema**). No difference exists between the formation of edema anywhere in the body except for the impact this edema has on gas exchange. In mild cases of pulmonary edema, a small decrease in arterial oxygenation can be detected. In severe cases, blood flow and ventilation are adversely affected with the potential for cardiopulmonary failure. The edema increases pulmonary vascular resistance, impedes gas diffusion, and induces bronchospasm once the fluid enters air space. Bronchospasm resulting from pulmonary edema is commonly referred to as **cardiac asthma**.

Common causes of pulmonary edema are

1. left ventricular failure with the consequential increase in pulmonary capillary pressure. This increase in pressure pushes more fluid out of the capillary bed into the interstitium, possibly even into the alveolar space.
2. leaky capillary membrane as a result of damage. Numerous diseases or physical trauma can damage the capillary membrane. Once damaged from physical insult such as inhalation of a toxic gas or invasion of a microorganism, the membrane becomes more permeable to fluid.
3. decreased plasma osmotic (colloid) pressure. Pulmonary capillary osmotic pressure is responsible for holding fluid inside the vessel. It is important to consider osmotic pressure in anemic patients.
4. fluid overload resulting from excessive administration of intravenous fluids. This situation increases hydrostatic pressure, pushing fluid into the interstitial space and possibly into the alveolus.
5. increased vascular resistance as a result of disease, which can have a dramatic effect on hydrostatic pressure. This also can cause the right ventricle to fail (cor pulmonale), further aggravating the problem.

Safety Factor

The most common cause of pulmonary edema is elevated pulmonary capillary pressure resulting from cardiac failure. Generally, capillary blood pressure must increase 2–3 mmHg above colloid osmotic pressure before edema develops. If normal capillary pressure is 8 mmHg and colloid osmotic pressure is 28 mmHg, there exists a safety factor of 23 mmHg against edema. When pressures are chronically elevated, lymphatic flow will be above normal levels to compensate for the fluid influx. Pulmonary lymphatics can enlarge and in-

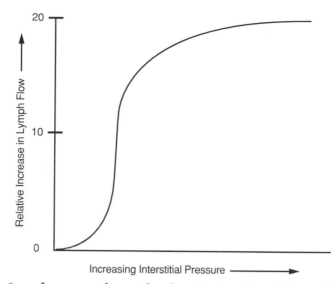

Figure 7-4. In pulmonary edema, the chronic elevation of interstitial pressure forces lymphatic flow to increase above normal levels to compensate for the influx of fluid.

crease flow as much as 20-fold above normal in chronic pulmonary hypertension (Figure 7-4).

▼ PULMONARY PRESSURES

Pulmonary pressures encompass a range of pressures from that found in the right ventricle to the pulmonary artery; to one from the pulmonary capillary bed; and, finally, to the pressure captured from the left atrium just before the blood enters the left ventricle. All of these pressures are depicted in Figure 7-5.

Right Ventricular Pressure

Pressure in the right ventricle ranges from a diastolic pressure (captured during muscle relaxation) of 0–1 mmHg to a systolic pressure of 25 mmHg. The extremely low pressure during diastole is necessary for refilling from the right atrium. Once the blood is pumped into the pulmonary artery (at a pressure of approximately 25 mmHg), it cannot return because of the pulmonic valve (semilunar valve). This is a one-way valve, which allows blood to travel out of the ventricle only.

Pulmonary Arterial Pressure

When the right ventricle contracts (systole), the pressure in the ventricle is essentially equal to the pressure in the pulmonary artery (i.e., approximately

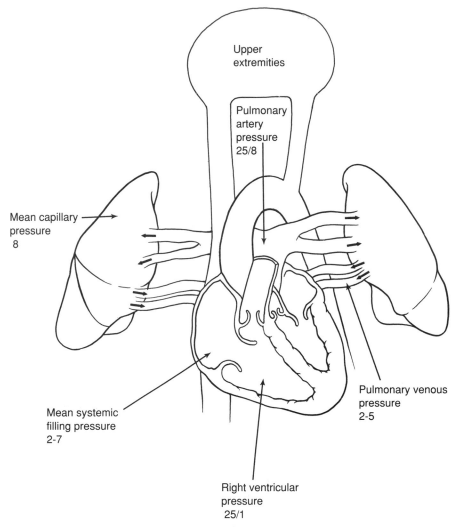

Figure 7-5.   Various cardiopulmonary pressures.

25 mmHg). However, when the right ventricle relaxes to allow refilling from the right atrium, the pulmonic valve closes and the pressure within the pulmonary artery remains above ventricular pressure. Pulmonary artery pressure begins to fill because blood is flowing through the capillaries, relieving the pressure. Because the blood is continually moving toward the left side of the heart, pressure would gradually decrease to zero if another right ventricular contraction did not occur.

Three major contributing factors to pulmonary artery blood pressures are

1. blood flow or cardiac output
2. vascular resistance or diameter of the pulmonary vasculature
3. pulmonary vascular compliance

Blood Flow or Cardiac Output (Right Ventricular)

As with airway pressure, if the resistance to flow remains constant and the flow is increased, pressure will increase correspondingly. Therefore, if pulmonary vascular resistance and/or compliance were to remain unchanged and cardiac output (ventricular blood volume output) increased, pressure would increase directly. The reverse is also true. Because flow is pulsatile (i.e., characterized by a rhythmic beat), pressure also is pulsatile. Cardiac output can be increased by either increased heart rate or stroke volume.

Pulmonary Vascular Resistance

The pulmonary arteries are surrounded by smooth muscle, which can constrict or relax in response to various stimuli. Again, if we compare the vasculature with the airways when flow remains constant, we see that pressures must increase as vascular caliber decreases. This resistance to blood flow is increased as vascular smooth muscle constricts and reduced as vascular smooth muscle relaxes:

Resistance to blood flow = [Mean pulmonary arterial pressure

— Pulmonary venous pressure]/Right ventricular blood flow

Alveolar **hypoxia** is characterized by decreased O_2 concentration in inspired air and is a potent constrictor of pulmonary vessel smooth muscle (hypoxic pulmonary vasoconstriction). The opposite also occurs: **hyperoxia** is an increase in O_2 concentration in the blood, leading to vasodilation. This response is extremely variable from one individual to another.

High levels of CO_2 also affect pulmonary smooth muscle. **Hypercapnia**, an increase in CO_2 in the blood, results in vascular constriction and a corresponding increase in pulmonary pressure.

The mechanism for the vascular response to hypoxia and hypercapnia is not well understood. However, their influence on blood flow and in selectively distributing blood to the better oxygenated and ventilated regions of the lung is an important compensatory mechanism in disease states.

Numerous other factors also can affect vascular smooth muscle tone in the lung, although in many cases the response is a mystery.

1. Histamine constricts only the pulmonary veins, not the arteries.
2. Many drugs and hormones cause inconsistent and variable responses from constriction to dilation.
3. Norepinephrine, epinephrine, and serotonin constrict both pulmonary arteries and veins.
4. Sympathetic stimulation and pulmonary embolism constrict arteries more than veins.
5. Generally, prostaglandins cause vasoconstriction, although some cause vasodilation, particularly those of the E series.
6. Acidosis causes pulmonary vasoconstriction and enhances hypoxic vasoconstriction.

TABLE 7-2 Pulmonary Vascular Tone	
Dilators	**Constrictors**
1. Beta agonists	1. Hypoxia
2. Anticholingeric	2. Hypercapnia
3. H_2 agonists	3. Acidosis
4. Acetylcholine	4. Sympathetic nerve stimulation
5. Bradykinin	5. Alpha agonists
6. Prostaglandins I_2 and E series	6. Serotonin
7. Theophylline	7. Angiotensin II
8. Nitric oxide	8. Prostaglandins F_{2alpha}, A_2, B_2
	9. Anaphylaxis
	10. Pulmonary embolism

Table 7-2 summarizes a series of factors that can either relax or contract pulmonary vascular smooth muscle. It is important to remember that elevated pulmonary arterial pressure increases right ventricular work. This increased work can result in cardiac rhythm irregularities and even cor pulmonale.

Pulmonary Vascular Compliance

The elastic properties of the pulmonary vasculature have a profound effect on pulmonary pressure. It should be remembered that the volumes of blood pumped through the lungs and systemic circulation are essentially equal. However, in the lungs the pressure is approximately one-fifth the systemic pressure. If it were not for the high compliance of the pulmonary vasculature, the ability of the system to absorb the blood volume would be significantly reduced and pulse pressure would be significantly increased (difference between systolic and diastolic pressure). The normal blood volume in the lungs is approximately 500 mL, about 10% of the total blood volume of the circulatory system. About 70 mL of this is actually in the capillaries and the rest is evenly distributed between the venous and arterial circulations. The ability of this system to expand and contract allows it to act as a reservoir. The volume of blood can be cut in half or doubled, depending on the physiological or pathological state.

Factors affecting pulmonary blood volume are as follows:

1. Increased thoracic pressure can have a significant effect on reducing blood volume.
2. Loss of blood from hemorrhage can be at least partially compensated for by a shift of blood from the lungs to the systemic circulation.
3. Mitral valve stenosis or regurgitation can result in a back pressure or damming up of blood volume, increasing the amount of blood reserved in the lungs. This inherent ability to respond allows the system to keep pressure relatively low under normal circumstances. When the system is overwhelmed, pulmonary edema may develop. This condition is said to occur when hydrostatic pressure that is pushing fluid out of the pulmonary capillary bed over-

whelms the osmotic pressure that is pulling fluid into the vascular space.

Pressures Surrounding the Pulmonary Vasculature

The pulmonary blood supply is surrounded by the air space of the lungs. Alveolar pressures are close to atmospheric pressure at ± 3 cm H_2O during normal spontaneous breathing. During forced inspiratory or expiratory maneuvers (i.e., coughing or sneezing) or during mechanical ventilation, these pressures can be considerably higher. This increase in pressure has a direct impact on the pulmonary vasculature. If the alveolar pressure is high enough, it can collapse the vessels. The pressure difference between the alveoli and the pulmonary vessel is commonly called transmural pressure. During maximum inspiration the radial traction pulling the lungs out has a significant impact on lowering transmural pressures. Arterial and venous calibers increase when the lung is spontaneously expanded.

The arteries and veins outside the alveolar regions act in a different manner. Because these vessels lay in the lung parenchyma, their calibers tend to respond to changes in lung volumes as they lay in the lung parenchyma. Vessels in the hilum and extending into the mediastinum are exposed to intrapleural pressures.

Pulmonary Pressure Monitoring

To monitor pulmonary artery pressure, a specialized flow-directed, balloon-tipped pulmonary artery catheter must be used (commonly called a Swan-Ganz catheter). The catheter is advanced through the right atrium into the right ventricle and on into the pulmonary artery. Eventually it wedges in a pulmonary artery and the balloon is deflated (Figure 7-6). Two openings allow for monitoring of central venous pressure and the pulmonary artery, as well as wedge pressure. It is useful in managing patients with

1. cardiogenic, hypovolemic, or septic shock
2. adult respiratory distress syndrome
3. pulmonary edema

In cardiovascular instability, fluid balance and ventricular function are difficult to monitor accurately without this catheter in place. The catheter may be placed in the basilic, brachial, femoral, subclavian, or internal jugular veins, although the latter two are the most commonly used placement sites. Typical pressures recorded from these readings are listed in Table 7-3.

Wedge Pressure

When the balloon is deflated, an opening in the distal tip of the catheter measures pulmonary artery pressure continuously, as well as systolic and diastolic pressures. Once the balloon is inflated, it measures pressures distal to the balloon, through the capillary bed. This measurement is referred to as pulmonary

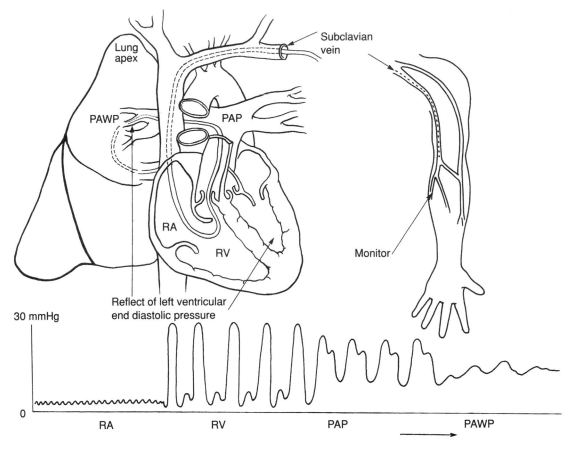

Figure 7-6.   A balloon catheter introduced into the right pulmonary artery captures PAWP.

TABLE 7-3 Pressure Measurements	
	Normal Range (mmHg)
Central venous pressure	2–10
Right atrial pressure	<10
Right ventricular systolic	15–30
Right ventricular diastolic	0–5
Pulmonary artery pressure	
Systolic	15–30
Diastolic	5–12
Mean	11–18
Mean pulmonary artery wedge pressure	5–12

artery wedge pressure (PAWP). It is a reflection of left ventricular preload or left ventricular end diastolic pressure, concepts described in Chapter 10.

▼ DISTRIBUTION OF BLOOD FLOW IN THE LUNGS

Under normal circumstances, the pulmonary vasculature is passive and responds to increased cardiac output or pressure by expanding. In actuality, when cardiac output increases during exercise, recruitment of vessels and expansion of the vasculature results in a decrease in pulmonary vascular resistance.

In an upright healthy individual blood flow is not evenly distributed throughout the lung. This variation may be a result of gravity, hypooxygenation, autonomic nervous control, exercise, or pathology.

Gravity

When a person is standing, the blood pressure can be 90 mmHg higher at the feet than it is at heart level. This difference results from the weight of the blood itself and is therefore dependent on gravity. Regardless of whether the person is supine, prone, or standing, the effect is always perpendicular to the ground.

The distance from the highest to the lowest point in a normal lung is approximately 30 cm. This translates to a 23 mmHg blood pressure difference between the base of the lung to its apex. The heart is situated about one third of the way up, leaving about 8 mmHg below and 15 mmHg above. This means that there is a pressure gain of about 8 mmHg in the base of the lung and a 15 mmHg pressure loss in the apex. This pressure difference has a dramatic effect on pulmonary blood flow.

The combination of this pressure decrease and the pressure that exists in the alveolus creates a variation in pulmonary perfusion. The most common model for describing this effect involves dividing the lung into zones 1–3.

Zone 1: Area of No Blood Flow
It is possible for pulmonary systolic and diastolic blood pressure to be lower than alveolar pressure. When this happens, the capillary is compressed and blood does not pass through (Figure 7-7). This creates a region of deadspace ventilation (ventilation of the alveolus without perfusion; see Chapter 8). This zone does not normally exist unless pulmonary blood pressure is abnormally reduced (i.e., through reduced cardiac output) or pulmonary alveolar pressure is abnormally increased (e.g., via mechanical ventilation).

Zone 2: Area of Pulsatile Blood Flow
In this area of the lung, pulmonary arteriole pressure is great enough to overcome the pressure in the alveolus during systole only (Figure 7-8). This area begins about 8 cm above the heart level and extends to the lung's apex.

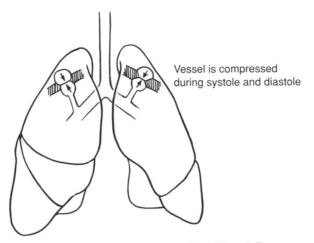

Vessel is compressed
during systole and diastole

Figure 7-7.   Zone 1: area of no blood flow.

Zone 3: Area of Continuous Blood Flow

From approximately 8 cm above the level of the heart down to the base of the lung is a region of continuous blood flow, in which both systolic and diastolic pressures are high enough to overcome alveolar pressure (Figure 7-9). In some of the lower regions of the lung, blood flow exceeds the amount of alveolar ventilation, resulting in inadequate gas exchange. This mismatching of ventilation and perfusion (V̇/Q̇) is referred to as the shunt effect, a term that will be discussed in detail in Chapter 8.

Hypooxygenation

Hypoxic pulmonary vasoconstriction is a term that describes the potent pulmonary vasculature–constricting effect of hypoxia. Hypoxia increases both pul-

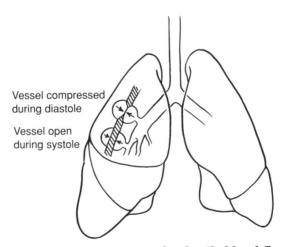

Vessel compressed
during diastole

Vessel open
during systole

Figure 7-8.   Zone 2: area of pulsatile blood flow.

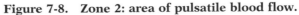

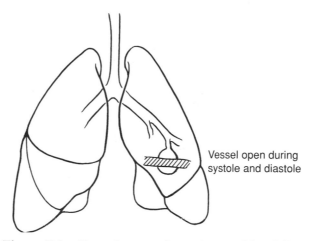

Figure 7-9.   Zone 3: area of continuous blood flow.

monary vascular resistance and pulmonary arterial pressure. Restoring O_2 levels causes vascular dilation, reducing pulmonary vascular resistance and pulmonary arterial pressure. The mechanism for this response is unknown, but it is partially responsible for the distribution of blood to the better oxygenated regions of the lung (Figure 7-10). (Blood is directed toward the well-oxygenated

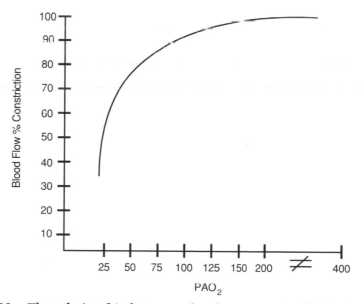

Figure 7-10.   The relationship between alveolar oxygen tension and pulmonary vascular smooth-muscle tone. As PAO$_2$ drops below 100 mmHg, the smooth muscle constricts to reduce blood flow to that region of the lung.

areas of the lung because its natural tendency is to follow the pathway of least resistance.) This helps ensure that blood matches with ventilation. In the case of pulmonary disease, ventilation may be unevenly distributed throughout the lung. To maximize gas exchange, blood flow is selectively distributed to areas with minimal disease.

Autonomic Nervous Control

Some nerves innervate lung tissue. However, it is doubtful that they play a significant role in the control of pulmonary blood flow. Vagal stimulation (10th cranial nerve) results in a small decrease in pulmonary vascular resistance. Sympathetic stimulation results in a small increase in pulmonary vascular resistance.

It is thought that the widespread vasoconstriction resulting from emboli occluding small pulmonary arteries is a result of a sympathetic reflex.

Exercise

During exercise the need to absorb larger volumes of O_2 (sometimes up to 20 times the normal uptake) is apparent. This increased absorption is accomplished in three ways:

1. Increasing the number of open capillaries to increase the amount of blood for gas exchange
2. Increasing cardiac output with increased blood flow through the lungs' picking up more O_2
3. Increasing alveolar ventilation, which increases the quantity of available O_2

Intrathoracic pressures and increased cardiac output can result in the entire lung becoming zone 3 (continuous blood flow throughout all lung fields).

Pathology

Many pathologic states can be responsible for obstruction or alteration of pulmonary blood flow. The following five common pathologies will be addressed: lung resection, pulmonary embolism, emphysema, pulmonary sclerosis, and atelectasis.

Lung Resection

If a lung is removed, pulmonary pressure is not increased because this is within the normal compensatory limits. However, the pulmonary reserve has been reduced significantly. Generally, problems do not arise as long as the individual remains inactive. When cardiac output begins to increase during exercise or stress, pulmonary pressures begin to increase rapidly, thus depleting the normal reserve. Diffusion capacity, the ability to exchange CO_2 and O_2 over a period of time, is significantly reduced.

Pulmonary Embolism

This is a thrombus (blood clot) or some other particulate matter that has become dislodged from somewhere in the body. When this object enters the lungs it becomes lodged in the capillary bed, the lung's natural filtering mechanism. It may occur as one large thrombus or a shower of smaller thrombi. Depending on the severity, this condition may result in blockage of pulmonary blood flow, pulmonary infarction, or tissue necrosis.

The affected region does not take part in gas exchange. This area is described as alveolar deadspace (ventilation without perfusion). Death may ensue if the embolus becomes large enough to tax the remaining vasculature beyond its limits (emboli have a tendency to grow once lodged). Humoral agents such as serotonin and prostaglandins are also released in response to the embolus. This results in bronchoconstriction and further aggravation of gas exchange capabilities by reduction of alveolar ventilation.

Emphysema

This disease is characterized by emphysematous cavities in place of many small alveoli. This results in a significant reduction in overall surface area and hence gas exchange capabilities. Both alveolar walls and vasculature are destroyed, progressively increasing pulmonary resistance and pulmonary artery pressure. Generalized alveolar hypoxia also results in hypoxic pulmonary vasoconstriction and a further increase in pulmonary vascular resistance. The generalized hypoxemia that results from this disease causes an increased cardiac output, further increasing pulmonary pressures and right ventricular work. Cor pulmonale is a common result. O_2 therapy can have a dramatic positive impact on patients with this disease.

Pulmonary Sclerosis

If the tissues or structures surrounding the pulmonary vasculature become fibrosed or stiff, pulmonary vascular compliance will be reduced. This reduction in the distensibility of the pulmonary vasculature results in a reduction in reserve. Pulmonary pressures may be normal at rest but increase significantly with even mild exercise.

Atelectasis

This collapse of alveolar units may involve a small part of the lung or may be widespread. It occurs when alveolar air is allowed to diffuse out into the blood without being replenished or if the lung is allowed to collapse as a result of pneumothorax (introduction of air into the thorax). The compression of pulmonary vasculature in combination with regional hypoxia significantly reduces blood flow into the area. If it is not too widespread, blood flow will simply be diverted to unaffected areas. *Selective redistribution of pulmonary blood flow* is a compensatory mechanism responsible for offsetting this condition.

A similar response can be seen with pneumonia or alveolar consolidation.

▼ METABOLIC FUNCTION OF THE LUNG

The lungs provide a number of important metabolic functions, including

1. the synthesis of phospholipids, a component of pulmonary surfactant.

2. protein synthesis, important for the formation of collagen and elastin in the structure of lung parenchyma.
3. metabolism of numerous vasoactive substances. For example, angiotensin I is converted to angiotensin II as it passes through the lungs. This potent vasoconstrictor is 50 times more active than its chemical precursor before entering the lung.
4. inactivation of numerous vasoactive substances as they pass through the lungs. Bradykinin and serotonin are for the most part inactivated as they pass through the lungs. This results from an uptake and storage process. Prostaglandin E_1, E_2, and F_{2alpha} are also inactivated in the lung.
5. the contribution of IgA, an immunoglobulin found in bronchial mucus, to the body's defense against microorganisms in the lungs.

▼ CONCLUSION

The pulmonary vasculature is a high-volume/low-pressure system. It can increase circulation three- to fivefold without significant increases in pulmonary vascular pressures. This reserve is necessary to accommodate the increased demands made during exercise and stress. In order to increase the absorption of O_2 and removal of CO_2, both blood supply and ventilation into the lung must be increased. Any disease condition that can hinder pulmonary blood supply in any way reduces the ability to exchange gas and hence reduces cardiopulmonary reserve.

❖ Review Questions

1. The systolic pressure created by the right side of the heart is (mmHg)
   a. 10.
   b. 25.
   c. 35.
   d. 80.
   e. 120.
2. The left atrium receives ——— pulmonary veins.
   a. 1
   b. 2
   c. 3
   d. 4
   e. 5
3. Lymphatic flow from the lung is approximately (mL/hr/100 g lung tissue)
   a. 1–2.
   b. 2–4.
   c. 5–6.

    d. 10–20.
    e. 18–26.
4. Lymphatic fluid moves through the lungs for the following reasons:
    i. lymphatic valves.
    ii. smooth muscle contraction and relaxation.
    iii. vessel compression.
    iv. changing systemic blood pressure.
    v. changing interstitial pH.

    a. i, ii, iii
    b. ii, iii, iv
    c. iii, iv, v
    d. i, ii, iii, iv
    e. All of the above

5. Pulmonary edema may be caused by
    i. left ventricular failure.
    ii. leaky capillary membrane.
    iii. decreased plasma osmotic pressure.
    iv. fluid overload.
    v. increased pulmonary blood pressure.

    a. i, ii, iii
    b. ii, iii, iv
    c. iii, iv, v
    d. i, ii, iii, iv
    e. All of the above

6. Three major contributing factors to pulmonary artery blood pressure are:
    i. systemic blood pressure.
    ii. lymphatic flow.
    iii. cardiac output.
    iv. pulmonary vascular resistance.
    v. pulmonary vascular compliance.

    a. i, ii, iii
    b. ii, iii, iv
    c. iii, iv, v
    d. i, iii, v
    e. ii, iv, v

7. Pulmonary vascular smooth muscle is constricted by
    i. hypoxia.
    ii. epinephrine.
    iii. hypercapnia.
    iv. acidosis.
    v. alpha agonists.

    a. i, ii, iii
    b. ii, iii, iv
    c. iii, iv, v

    d. ii, iii, iv, v

    e. All of the above

8. Pulmonary vascular smooth muscle dilation results from

    i. beta agonists.

    ii. hypoxia.

    iii. anticholinergics.

    iv. acidosis.

    v. theophylline.

    a. i, ii, iii

    b. ii, iii, iv

    c. iii, iv, v

    d. i, iii, v

    e. All of the above

9. Which of the following statements describes Zone 3 in the lungs?

    a. $P_{Alveolar}$ > Pulmonary capillary systolic > Pulmonary capillary diastolic

    b. Pulmonary capillary systolic > $P_{Alveolar}$ > Pulmonary capillary diastolic

    c. Pulmonary capillary systolic and diastolic pressure > $P_{Alveolar}$

    d. Pulmonary alveolar pressure > Pulmonary vascular pressure

    e. $P_{Alveolar}$ < Systemic blood pressure < Pulmonary blood pressure

Data for calculations in questions 10, 11, 12.

		10	11	12
(mmHg)	PaO_2	100	80	70
(mmHg)	$PaCO_2$	40	45	47
(mL/dL)	$CaCO_2$	49	50	51
(mL/dL)	CaO_2	20	19	18
(mL/dL)	$C\bar{v}O_2$	15	14	13
(mL/dL)	CcO_2	21	21	20

10. Given the information listed in column 10, calculate the physiological shunt.

    a. 13%

    b. 17%

    c. 28.6%

    d. 32.5%

    e. 41.3%

11. Given the information listed in column 11, calculate the physiological shunt.

    a. 16.5%

    b. 17.2%

    c. 28.6%

    d. 31.5%

    e. 41.3%

12. Given the information listed in column 12, calculate the physiological shunt.
    a. 13%
    b. 17%
    c. 28.6%
    d. 32.5%
    e. 42.5%

8

VENTILATION–PERFUSION RELATIONSHIPS

OBJECTIVES

1. Describe deadspace.
2. Discuss the deadspace effect.
3. Describe a shunt effect.
4. Define true shunting.
5. Address the concept of physiological shunt.
6. Reiterate the shunt equation.
7. Detail how the impact of intrapulmonary shunting can be minimized.
8. Describe the oxygen cascade.

Matthews LR: CARDIOPULMONARY ANATOMY AND PHYSIOLOGY. © 1996 Lippincott–Raven Publishers.

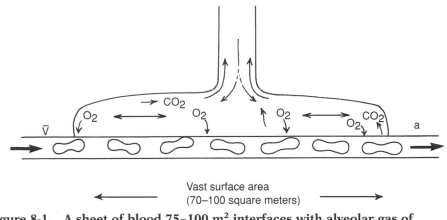

Vast surface area
(70–100 square meters)

Figure 8-1.   A sheet of blood 75–100 m² interfaces with alveolar gas of approximately the same dimensions. If the two surfaces do not match up, diffusion is impaired.

This chapter uses many of the physiological concepts discussed in the preceding chapters as the foundation for a discussion of matching blood and gas in the lung. When we consider the impact of a disease condition on the cardiopulmonary system, it is often the ventilation/perfusion ($\dot{V}/\dot{Q}$) relationship that we are concerned about because of its direct impact on gas exchange.

Thus far we have considered ventilation, diffusion, and perfusion. When everything is functioning adequately, synchronization of all of these processes results in adequate gas exchange and leaves a considerable reserve to meet the demands of stress and exercise. Figure 8-1 shows the ideal relationship between ventilation and perfusion. It is only when the surface area of blood fails to match up with that of alveolar gas that diffusion is impaired. Because the mismatching of ventilation and perfusion is responsible for the vast majority of gas exchange disturbances in pulmonary disease, we will examine this relationship in detail.

There are five possible $\dot{V}/\dot{Q}$ relationships that can exist in the lung:

1. Deadspace (V_D) ventilation (ratio 1:0)
2. V_D effect (ratio 1:0.5, high or increased)
3. One-to-one $\dot{V}/\dot{Q}$ matching (1:1)
4. Shunt effect (ratio 1:2, low or decreased)
5. True shunt (ratio 1:0)

▼ DEADSPACE VENTILATION

Remember, physiological V_D is the sum of alveolar V_D and physiological V_D:

$$\text{Physiological } V_D = \text{alveolar } V_D + \text{anatomical } V_D$$

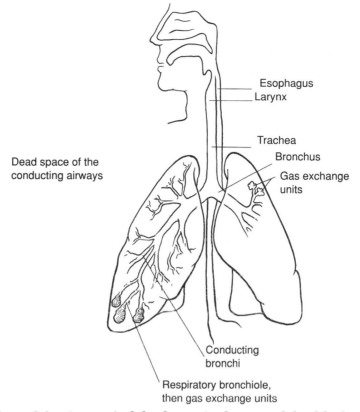

Esophagus
Larynx

Trachea
Bronchus
Gas exchange units

Dead space of the
conducting airways

Conducting
bronchi

Respiratory bronchiole,
then gas exchange units

Figure 8-2.   Anatomical deadspace in the normal, healthy lung.

In a normal, healthy lung anatomical V_D exists at the connecting ducts that lead into the gas exchange units (Figure 8-2). The normal value of this anatomical V_D, which plays no part in gas exchange, is approximately 1 mL/lb, or 2.0 mL/kg, ideal body weight.

Alveolar Deadspace

The absence of blood flow into an alveolus (lack of perfusion) results in wasted ventilation. This wasted ventilation is referred to as **alveolar deadspace**. Normally, this does not exist in a healthy lung.

There are two primary pathological reasons for the development of V_D:

1. Decreased cardiac output or pulmonary hypotension
2. Pulmonary embolus

Decreased Cardiac Output or Pulmonary Hypotension

As cardiac output or pulmonary blood pressure is decreased, the amount of wasted ventilation increases. More and more functional lung units lose their blood supply, and the ventilation entering that region is wasted. Anything that adversely affects the right ventricle's ability to perfuse the lung impacts on the amount of alveolar V_D. In the upright lung, the uppermost lung regions are poorly perfused relative to the bases, a concept described later in this chapter.

Because this gas is not involved with gas exchange, it enters and exits the lung unit with the same gas concentration (Figure 8-3a). Therefore, exhaled gas concentrations from an alveolar V_D region are essentially equivalent to those in room air. The partial pressure of oxygen (O_2) in the alveoli (PAO_2) is approximately 150 mmHg; partial pressure of carbon dioxide (CO_2) in the alveoli ($PACO_2$) is approximately 0.0 mmHg. This gas exits the lung and dilutes the exhaled gases coming from lung units involved in gas diffusion. Remember that arterial partial pressure of CO_2 ($PaCO_2$) is normally very close to end-tidal CO_2 ($P_{ET}CO_2$). The alveolar V_D dilution of this gas puts a larger difference between $P_{ET}CO_2$ and $PaCO_2$. Alveolar V_D is calculated by subtracting anatomical V_D from physiological V_D.

$$\text{Alveolar } V_D = \text{physiological } V_D - \text{anatomical } V_D$$

Another more convenient, although possibly less accurate, method of estimating alveolar V_D is:

$$\text{Alveolar } V_D = [PaCO_2 - P_{ET}CO_2] / PaCO_2$$

An end-tidal CO_2 monitor can be used as an indicator of the effectiveness of cardiopulmonary resuscitation (CPR). As end-tidal CO_2 increases, CPR effectiveness increases; the reverse is also true.

Pulmonary Embolus

This condition results in the blockage of blood flow into the pulmonary vasculature. The same disruption occurs in terms of gas exchange as described above. As the embolus increases in size, the difference between end-tidal CO_2 and arterial PCO_2 begins to increase (end-tidal CO_2 decreases). A significant pulmonary embolism results in pulmonary hypertension and bronchospasm, causing major disruptions in $\dot{V}/\dot{Q}$ relationships.

▼ DEADSPACE EFFECT

The V_D effect is an area of hyperventilation that is characterized as follows:

$$\text{Hyperventilation} \rightarrow \text{increased } \dot{V}/\dot{Q}$$

In this condition, ventilation is in excess of perfusion (Figure 8-3b). It is not entirely wasted, but it exceeds the amount of perfusion ($PAO_2 > 100$ mmHg $PaCO_2 < 35$ mmHg) and results in a decreased $P_{ET}CO_2$ and the average exhaled CO_2 ($PECO_2$).

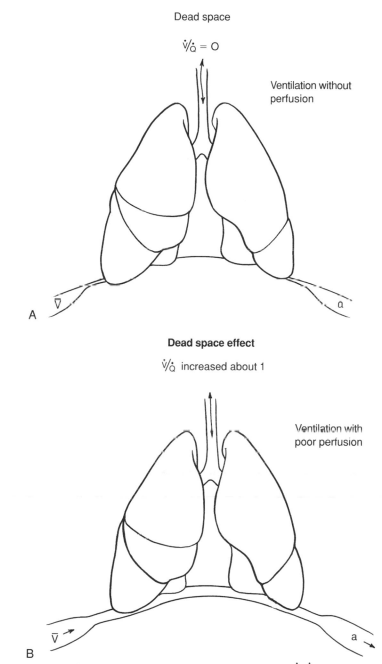

Dead space

$\dot{V}/\dot{Q} = O$

Ventilation without perfusion

A $\overline{v}$ a

Dead space effect

$\dot{V}/\dot{Q}$ increased about 1

Ventilation with poor perfusion

$\overline{V}$ a

B

Figure 8-3. Deadspace (a), deadspace effect (b), $1:1$ $\dot{V}/\dot{Q}$ (c), shunt effect (d), and true shunt (e).

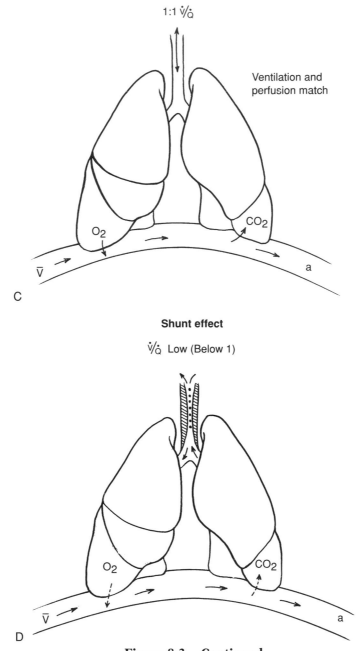

Shunt effect

$\dot{V}/\dot{Q}$ Low (Below 1)

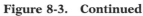

Figure 8-3.   Continued

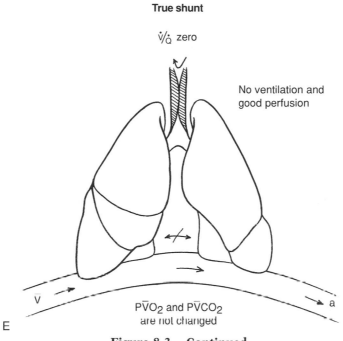

Figure 8-3. Continued

▼ ONE-TO-ONE VENTILATION/PERFUSION MATCHING

In this case both blood flow and ventilation are matched. Equilibration between alveolar gas and blood occurs and the two components are in balance (Figure 8-3c). PAO_2 is approximately 100 mmHg and $PACO_2$ is approximately 40 mmHg.

The amount of CO_2 liberated and O_2 absorbed (**respiratory exchange ratio**) is in balance with CO_2 produced and O_2 consumed at a cellular level (**respiratory quotient**). If this ideal state occurred throughout both lungs, PAO_2 would be equal to the arterial partial pressure of O_2 (PaO_2). The only difference between the two values would be the result of a diffusion difference across the alveolar–capillary (A/C) membrane (Oswald partition coefficient) and anatomical shunting.

See Figure 8-4 for a complete description of the ventilation/perfusion relationship in the lung.

▼ SHUNT EFFECT

The **shunt effect** creates a region of higher perfusion than ventilation, which causes blood to leave the lung before gas exchange is complete (Figure 8-3d). The blood is thus hypoventilated, with $PaO_2 < 90$ mmHg $PaCO_2 > 40$ mmHg:

Hypoventilation − Decreased $\dot{V}/\dot{Q}$ (ratio $1:2$)

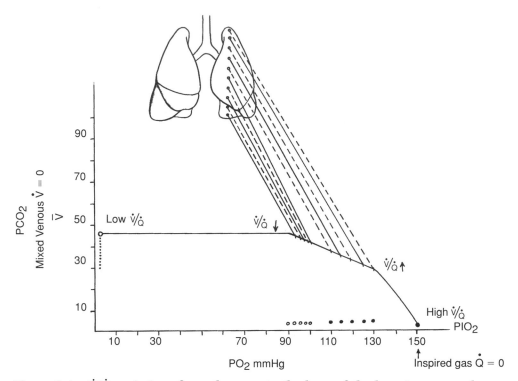

Figure 8-4.   V̇/Q̇ variations from the apex to the base of the lung in a normal upright individual.

The shunt effect exists to a small degree in the base of even the healthiest lung. This condition causes a slight decrease in arterial O_2 content (1–3% of the normal physiological shunt), which is described in an upcoming section.

If mucus, bronchospasm, edema, or exudate interferes with ventilation, a shunt effect can occur in one or more regions of the lung. The bronchospasm or hypersecretions increase airway resistance and reduce the flow of gas into a region of the lung. Because gas flow always follows the pathway of least resistance, areas with low resistance are better ventilated than are areas of higher resistance. Generally, ventilation favors the healthier regions of the lung. This results in an uneven distribution of ventilation and therefore an uneven exchange of gases from one area to another. Not all of the blood passing through the lungs is adequately oxygenated and ventilated. As a result, CO_2 and O_2 pressures are close to venous levels when the blood leaves a region that is poorly ventilated. When this blood mixes with well-ventilated blood, PaO_2 is decreased and $PaCO_2$ is increased. The addition of venous blood to arterial blood is known as a **venous admixture**.

There are a number of other factors that lead to hypoventilation:

1. Central nervous system depressant drugs (i.e., morphine and barbiturates)

2. Chest wall damage (i.e., flail chest)
3. Respiratory muscle paralysis
5. True shunt (capillary shunting)

A true shunt develops in a region of the lung where there is perfusion but no ventilation (Figure 8-3e). In the absence of ventilation, either consolidation (filling of the alveolus with fluid and/or particulate matter) or atelectasis results. Blood flows from the right side of the heart through the pulmonary arteries into the capillary bed, then through the pulmonary vein, and back into the left side of the heart without exchanging gas. This is a true venous admixture. Venous blood enters the left ventricle, diluting arterial blood, reducing PaO_2, and increasing $PaCO_2$ (venous blood is low in O_2 and high in CO_2). It is important to remember that this venous blood does not come in contact with a ventilated alveolus.

O_2 therapy has little impact on arterial oxygenation, a condition known as refractory **hypoxemia**.

Anatomical Shunting

A normal anatomical shunt exists in the body and is used for routing venous blood directly into arterial blood. This anatomical shunting is achieved through the following structures:

1. Thebesian veins
2. Bronchial circulation
3. Pleural circulation

Thebesian Veins

A small portion of the coronary blood drainage is achieved through the thebesian veins, which are venules that carry blood from the myocardium to the atria or ventricles. The coronary blood empties directly into the left ventricle, where its decreased PaO_2 and increased $PaCO_2$ qualify it as a venous admixture. Coronary circulation primarily empties back into the right ventricle, but a small portion of it empties into the pulmonary veins and, therefore, the left ventricle. This also becomes a venous admixture (decreased PaO_2 and increased $PaCO_2$).

Bronchial Circulation

About 1–2% of cardiac output is received by the bronchial circulation. It supplies the supporting tissues of the lungs with O_2 and nutrients. Once it has exchanged with the tissues, it empties back into the left atrium, and then to the left ventricle. This results in a venous admixture, characterized by a corresponding decrease in PaO_2 and an increase in $PaCO_2$.

Pleural Circulation

This system supplies the visceral pleura with O_2 and nutrients. It also drains into the left side of the heart and likewise results in a venous admixture with the corresponding decrease in PaO_2 and increase in $PaCO_2$.

The combination of thebesian, bronchial, and pleural circulations accounts for a combined anatomical shunt of 1–3% of cardiac output.

Physiological Shunt

This is the combined total of all forms of shunt, both capillary and anatomical. It accounts for 2–6% of the total cardiac output. Anatomical shunt remains unchanged in health and disease. Therefore, in the absence of cardiac or vascular anomalies, any increase in physiological shunt results from capillary shunting in the lung. This means that under most circumstances intrapulmonary shunting can be measured by measuring physiological shunting. The measurement is an indication of how much blood is or is not taking part in gas exchange.

Measurement of Physiological Shunt

Ideally, all blood that leaves the right ventricle enters the left ventricle oxygenated and ventilated, resulting in a PaO_2 of approximately 100 mmHg and a $PaCO_2$ of approximately 40 mmHg. There would not be venous blood mixing with arterial blood from capillary or anatomical shunting. We know this does not occur in reality. In fact, PaO_2 is lower than ideal and $PaCO_2$ is higher than ideal. If we calculate the alveolar PO_2 and measure the arterial PO_2, the difference between the two values should be an indication of how much shunt, both capillary and anatomical, is present. Calculating the amount of shunted blood in comparison with the total cardiac output provides us with a numerical value that indicates the amount of total cardiac output that is shunted blood. This is expressed mathematically as follows:

$$°Q_S/°Q_T \times 100$$

where $°Q_S$ is the cardiac output that is shunted (does not take part in gas exchange) and $°Q_T$ is the total cardiac output, both shunted and not shunted (the total cardiac output is all of the blood that exits the ventricle.) This includes that which takes part in gas exchange and that which does not.

This formula gives the amount of shunted blood as a percentage of the total cardiac output. As described above, $°Q_S$ refers to the cardiac output that is shunted. Therefore, it is indicative of the difference between ideal and actual content of O_2 in the blood.

Ideal Oxygen Content in the Blood

The ideal content of O_2 in blood is commonly expressed as CIO_2, although it may be written as CCO_2 (content of capillary O_2). This value is calculated as follows:

$$CIO_2 = (PAO_2 \times 0.003) + (1.34 \times Hb)$$

This equation can be described in two parts, as shown below:

Part 1   Part 2

$$PAO_2 = [(P_{Barometric} - 47) \times FIO_2] - [PaCO_2(FIO_2 + 1 - FIO_2)]/R$$

Part 1: Because alveolar gas is 100% saturated with water and is normally 37°C, the water vapor pressure is 47 mmHg. It must be subtracted from the total barometric pressure before a partial pressure for gas can be calculated. If the FIO_2 (fractional inspired O_2 concentration) is 0.21, or 21% (O_2 occupies 21% of the total gas pressure dry), we then multiply 0.21 by the barometric pressure to get the partial pressure of O_2.

Part 2: O_2 is continuously being removed from alveolar gas. When the respiratory exchange ratio is 0.8, approximately 20% more O_2 is being removed from the alveolus than CO_2 is being replaced. Because alveolar CO_2 partial pressure is close to arterial CO_2 partial pressure, it is a substitute for $PACO_2$. Dividing by the respiratory exchange ratio fraction approximates the partial pressure of O_2 being removed from the alveolar gas. When this pressure is subtracted from the partial pressure of O_2 in ambient gas, alveolar O_2 pressure is represented.

Ideal Arterial Oxygen Pressure

The ideal PaO_2 is equal to alveolar pressure. In the absence of physiological shunt, arterial O_2 pressure would be equal to alveolar O_2 pressure. Therefore, any difference between alveolar and arterial O_2 pressure would approximate physiological shunting.

The ideal partial pressure of O_2 is converted to content in arterial blood when it is multiplied by the solubility coefficient for O_2 (0.003 mL O_2/mmHg/100 mL of blood at 37°C).

This content, which is dissolved in plasma, is added to the ideal amount of O_2 being carried by hemoglobin. If the hemoglobin molecule is 100% saturated (full of O_2), it carries 1.34 mL of O_2 for every gram of hemoglobin.

Actual Content of Oxygen in Arterial Blood

As we have seen, the actual O_2 content of blood does not necessarily equal the ideal O_2 content. The actual content is measured using the following equation:

$$\text{Part 1} \qquad\qquad \text{Part 2}$$
$$(PaO_2 \times 0.003) + (1.34 \times Hb \times Sata)$$

Part 1 indicates the volume of O_2 being carried in the arterial plasma. PaO_2 represents the partial pressure of O_2 in arterial blood. It is a measured, as opposed to calculated, value, derived from drawing an arterial sample from the patient and analyzing blood gas in a polarographic O_2 electrode. It is then converted to content by multiplying this measured value by the solubility coefficient of O_2 (0.003 mL/mmHg/100 mL of blood at 37°C).

$$PaO_2 \times 0.003 = \text{content of } O_2 \text{ in arterial blood (in milliliters)}$$
$$\text{per 100 mL blood (carried in solution only)}$$

In Part 2, the volume of O_2 being carried by hemoglobin (Hb) in arterial blood is represented as follows:

$$1.34 \times Hb \times Sata$$

where 1.34 is the number of milliliters of O_2 carried by 1 g of hemoglobin when it is 100% full, and Hb is the hemoglobin value in grams per 100 mL of blood.

Saturation of arterial blood ($Sata$) is the measurement of an actual amount of O_2 carried by the Hb compared with the amount that could be carried if the Hb were 100% full. Arterial blood is introduced into a spectrophotometer, and measurements are taken of the total Hb and the O_2-carrying Hb content of blood (these SI units are grams per liter). These measurements are expressed as a percentage.

The amount of Hb available to carry O_2 is calculated as follows:

%Saturation of O_2 in Hb = arterial blood/total Hb in blood

$CIO_2 - CaO_2$

The difference between ideal and actual O_2 content in blood is an indication of the amount of shunting taking place. If there were no shunting, the actual O_2 content would be equal to the ideal O_2 content because all of the blood would become 100% saturated with O_2. With 100% shunting (i.e., no gas exchange taking place in the lung), the venous blood would eventually have nearly a 0% O_2 content.

$CaO_2 - C\bar{v}O_2$

$C\bar{v}O_2$ is the content of O_2 in mixed venous blood returning from all body systems. This blood sample is best taken from the pulmonary artery via a pulmonary artery catheter (Figure 7.6).

$$C\bar{v}O_2 = (1.34 \times Hg \times Sat\bar{v}) + (0.003 \times P\bar{v}O_2)$$

The difference between the O_2 content of arterial and venous blood is determined by whether O_2 is being added to or taken away from the blood during gas exchange. In the lung, O_2 is added to the mixed venous blood and the blood becomes arterialized, or oxygenated. Therefore, this value is an indication of the amount of blood that is exchanged with gas. More simply put, it is the amount of blood that is not shunted.

Therefore,

$$\dot{Q}_S/\dot{Q}_T = \frac{\overset{\text{(shunted blood)}}{(CIO_2 - CaO_2)}}{\underset{\text{(shunted blood)   (unshunted blood)}}{(CIO_2 - CaO_2) + (CaO_2 - C\bar{v}O_2)}}$$

is

Shunted blood/total blood (shunted and unshunted)

Multiplying this decimal by 100 yields the percentage of shunted blood compared with total cardiac output.

Mixed Venous Oxygen Content

By the time the blood is pumped out of the right side of the heart, it has returned from all parts of the body with an average O_2 content of approximately

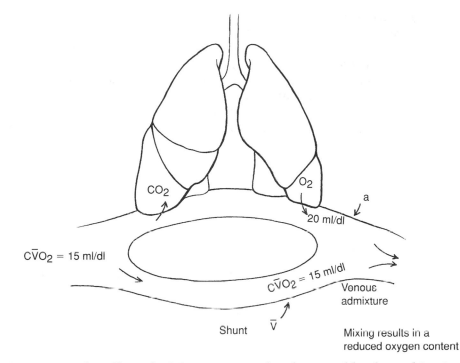

Figure 8-5. The effect of mixing oxygenated and venous blood, resulting in an overall reduction in oxygen content.

15 mL/100 mL of blood. It should be remembered that blood returning from different organ systems has different quantities of O_2 remaining in it. This is why all of the blood must be mixed together and equilibration must take place before measurements of samples can be used in the shunt equation (Figure 8.5).

$\dot{Q}_S$ SHUNT

Because this blood bypasses ventilated regions of the lung, it does not gain O_2 or liberate CO_2. This blood returns to the left side of the heart with O_2 and CO_2 contents the same as that of mixed venous blood (venous admixture). It reduces the O_2 content and increases the CO_2 content of blood entering the left side of the heart (Figure 8.5).

$\dot{Q}_T$ TOTAL CARDIAC OUTPUT

This is the blood that has been mixed from all regions of the lung as well as from anatomical shunting. As the quantity of shunted blood increases, the content of O_2 in the blood returning to the left side of the heart decreases (Figure 8.5).

Minimizing the Impact of Intrapulmonary Shunting

When a disease process impedes or stops gas flow to a region of the lung, intrapulmonary shunting develops. As a result, particular attention must be directed to maintaining a satisfactory cardiac output. An increase or decrease in cardiac output can have a dramatic impact on the significance of a specific size shunt. When cardiac output is decreased, more O_2 must be removed from a given volume of blood (if O_2 consumption remains the same). Therefore, if mixed venous O_2 content is decreased and this increases the impact, a shunt has an arterial O_2 content. Both the size of a shunt and the amount of O_2 in mixed venous blood impact on arterial O_2 content.

For example, normal values for O_2 content and saturation are as follows:

$$CaO_2 = 20 \text{ mL/dL arteriovenous}$$

$$C\bar{v}O_2 = 15 \text{ mL/dL difference of 5 mL/dL}$$

$$\dot{Q}_S/\dot{Q}_T = \sim5\%$$

Examples of Shunting

Example #1

In order to simplify calculations, if we assume unshunted blood becomes 100% saturated, then the following is true:

1. 95% of the cardiac output exits the lung with 20 mL of O_2 per 100 mL of blood.
2. 5% of the cardiac output exits the lung with the same content as mixed venous blood, 15 mL of O_2 per 100 mL of blood.
3. The 95% with 20 vol/dL mixes with 5% of 15 mL/dL, yielding the following results:

$$0.95 \times 20 = 19.0$$
$$0.05 \times 15 = 0.75$$
Arterial O_2 content $= 19.75$ mL/100 mL of blood

If 100% of the blood received 20 vol/dL of O_2, the resulting arterial O_2 content would be 20 vol/dL. Therefore,

$19.75/20.00 = 0.99$, or 99%

4. This shows us that with a 5% shunt and a mixed venous content of 15 vol/dL, arterial blood would fall 1% short of the ideal content.

Example #2

What would happen if this same individual were to inhale a foreign object that lodged in a main bronchus, creating a 30% shunt? The following predictable steps would occur:

1. Suddenly the percentage of blood leaving the lungs to enter the left side of the heart would increase from 5% to 30%; furthermore, it would contain 15 mL/dL of O_2 (mixed venous O_2 content).
2. This increased venous admixture will result in a decreased arterial O_2 content, calculated as follows:

$$0.7 \times 20 = 14.0$$
$$0.3 \times 15 = 4.5$$
$$\text{Arterial content} = 18.5 \text{ mL/dL}$$
$$18.5/20 = 0.93, \text{ or } 93\%$$

Arterial blood has decreased from 99% to 93% of its ideal value.

Example #3

If O_2 consumption and cardiac output remain unchanged, the arterial venous difference is still 5 mL/dL. This significantly reduces the end-point arterial venous content. Its normal difference is a value of 5 mL/dL (19.75 to 14.75). After occluding the bronchi, the arterial content will decrease from 18.50 mL/dL to a mixed venous content of 13.50 mL/dL.

As a result, mixed venous blood has an O_2 content of 13.5 mL/dL. If the shunt remains at 30%, a further impact will result. The resulting arterial content will equal the sum of unshunted and shunted blood:

Unshunted: $0.7 \times 20.0 - 14.0$
Shunted: $0.3 \times 13.5 - 4.1$
Total: 18.1
or $18.1/20 - 90\%$

Arterial blood thus carries 10% less of what it could be carrying if it were full.

Arterial blood, which originally had decreased from 99% down to 93%, has further decreased to 90% because of the decrease in mixed venous O_2 content.

It can easily be seen that this vicious cycle could continue if the normal compensatory mechanisms did not work together in an attempt to minimize this physiological insult.

1. Increased cardiac output is the most important compensatory mechanism for hypoxemia. When cardiac output increases, provided O_2 consumption remains unchanged, mixed venous O_2 content increases. This increased cardiac output increases O_2 delivery to the tissues and reduces the impact of the shunt.
2. Selective distribution of blood flow to the better oxygenated and ventilated regions of the lung also diverts blood away from the affected area in the lung. Remember that acidosis and hypoxemia are both pulmonary vasoconstrictors.

Increased Oxygen Consumption

If O_2 consumption is increased for any reason (i.e., increased body temperature, seizures, work of breathing) and cardiac output does not increase, correspondingly mixed venous O_2 content will decrease. This decrease in mixed venous O_2 content may aggravate any existing pulmonary limitations (Figure 8-4).

It is worth noting that increasing cardiac output to increase mixed venous oxygen content may cause dilation of the vasculature in the shunt regions of the lung. This partially offsets the benefit of increasing cardiac output by increasing the total volume of shunted blood.

Diffusion and Perfusion Limitations

The time it takes for a red blood cell (RBC) to pass through the pulmonary capillary bed is about 0.75 seconds. PaO_2 is essentially equal to PAO_2 when the RBC is one third of the way through its contact with alveolar air. When cardiac output is markedly increased, as in exercise, the time an RBC spends in the gas exchange region may be reduced by one third. However, gas exchange is still adequate with little or no decrease in arterial PO_2. Reduced alveolar PO_2, a diffusion barrier, and perfusion limitation can all limit the transfer of O_2 into the blood. One should remember that the capacity of the RBC to absorb O_2 rapidly accounts for the rapid uptake of O_2 as the RBC enters the pulmonary capillary bed. Without hemoglobin in the RBC, equilibration would occur, but the O_2-carrying capacity would be insufficient to sustain life.

▼ CONCLUSION

In this chapter we explored the various $\dot{V}/\dot{Q}$ relationships and their roles in enhancing or obstructing cardiopulmonary function. As we saw in the last section, perfusion (and hence ventilation) depends on the RBC's ability to diffuse through the pulmonary capillary bed unimpeded by anatomical or physiological obstructions. The RBC's role in gas transport is so central to adequate $\dot{V}/\dot{Q}$ relationships that it deserves a chapter of its own.

❖ Review Questions

1. Deadspace is indicative of a $\dot{V}/\dot{Q}$ of
   i. $1:1$.
   ii. $0.5:1$.
   iii. $2:1$.
   iv. $1:3$
   v. $3:1$.

   a. i, ii
   b. i, iv
   c. iii, v
   d. i, iii, v
   e. i, ii, iv

2. Alveolar deadspace results from
   i.   decreased cardiac output.
   ii. pulmonary embolus.

iii. increased cardiac output.

iv. pneumothorax.

v. pneumonia.

a. ii, iii

b. i, ii

c. ii, iii, iv

d. iii, iv, v

e. ii, iv, v

3. In pulmonary embolus,

i. end-tidal CO_2 to arterial CO_2 increases.

ii. end-tidal CO_2 is increased.

iii. bronchospasm results.

iv. preload is reduced.

v. pulmonary hypertension may result.

a. i, ii, iii

b. ii, iii, iv

c. i, iii, v

d. iii, iv, v

e. i, iii, iv, v

4. In pneumonia,

i. true shunting occurs.

ii. end-tidal CO_2 is decreased.

iii. cardiac output is increased.

iv. pulmonary hypotension results.

v. $\dot{V}/\dot{Q}$ is decreased.

a. ii, iii, iv

b. iii, iv, v

c. i, iii, iv

d. i, iii, v

e. ii, iv, v

5. Normal physiologic anatomical shunting results from

i. thebesian veins.

ii. bronchial circulation.

iii. pleural circulation.

iv. stasis atelectasis.

v. ventilation/perfusion mismatching.

a. i, iii, v

b. ii, iii, iv

c. i, ii, iii

d. i, iii, iv

e. iii, iv, v

9

GAS TRANSPORT AND THE RED BLOOD CELL

OBJECTIVES

1. Describe the various methods by which oxygen is carried in the blood.

2. Formulate Henry's law.

3. Define affinity.

4. Describe P_{50}.

5. Examine the various factors responsible for a shift of the oxyhemoglobin dissociation curve.

Matthews LR: CARDIOPULMONARY ANATOMY AND PHYSIOLOGY. © 1996 Lippincott–Raven Publishers.

6. Set forth the various factors responsible for a shift of the carbon dioxide dissociation curve.

7. Discuss the various methods by which carbon dioxide is carried in the blood.

8. Explore the effect blood flow has on interstitial fluid PO_2 (mmHg).

9. Describe the effect blood flow has on interstitial fluid PCO_2 (mmHg).

10. Describe the hemoglobin molecule.

11. Identify the normal values for hemoglobin.

12. List and characterize abnormalities in gas transport.

The average person uses 250 mL of oxygen (O_2) every minute and produces 200 mL of carbon dioxide (CO_2). Continuous and uninterrupted transport of these exchanged gases is essential for life. Inspired O_2 must be carried from the lungs out into the tissues, and CO_2 must be carried from the tissues back to the lungs for expulsion into the atmosphere. A complex set of chemical and physical reactions allows this to occur. In the absence of the red blood cell (RBC, or erythrocyte) and its specialized function, sufficient quantities of CO_2 and O_2 could not be carried. This chapter describes the various mechanisms by which O_2 and CO_2 are carried in the blood.

RBCs are produced in the bone marrow and function for approximately 120 days. Once damaged or nonfunctional, they are destroyed by *phagocytes* (cells that ingest and destroy particulate matter) in the spleen, liver, and red bone marrow. In this process, iron is salvaged and returned to the bone marrow to produce new hemoglobin. Regulation of RBC concentrations in the blood, within very narrow ranges, is essential. Abnormalities in RBCs or hemoglobin concentration can significantly impair the blood's O_2-carrying capacities, scenarios that will be addressed later in this chapter (see "Abnormalities in Gas Transport").

▼ OXYGEN TRANSPORT

O_2 is carried in the blood in two forms: it is either dissolved in plasma or combined with hemoglobin inside the RBC.

Oxygen Dissolved and Carried in Plasma

Only a small portion of O_2 is actually carried dissolved in plasma (2–4%), but this is the medium for transport of O_2 back and forth between the lung and RBCs, as well as between the RBCs and the tissues. As mixed venous blood enters the lung, its partial O_2 pressure ($P\bar{v}O_2$) is low, approximately 40 mmHg, and alveolar PO_2 (PAO_2) is approximately 100 mmHg. O_2 moves rapidly into the blood in response to a pressure gradient. The plasma absorbs 0.003 mL of O_2 per 100 mL of blood per mmHg pressure at 37°C. A simple calculation shows that at an arterial O_2 pressure (PaO_2) of 100 mmHg (100×0.003 mL/100 mL of blood/mmHg at 37°C), the blood carries only 0.3 mL of O_2 per 100 mL of blood. This accounts for only a small percentage of the O_2 required to maintain normal basal metabolic functions. Normally, 5 mL of O_2 is used from every 100 mL of blood. Remember, however, that the plasma (the liquid portion of blood) is an essential medium for transport of gases into and out of the bloodstream.

Example #1

If the total amount of O_2 used per 100 mL of blood is 5 mL and PaO_2 decreases from 100 mmHg to 40 mmHg after it passes through the capillary bed, what percentage of O_2 used comes from the plasma?

Solving this problem requires that we follow two sequential computational steps:

1. *Calculate the amount of O_2 used.* A decrease from 100 mmHg down to 40 mmHg is a decrease of 60 mmHg. If the blood carries 0.003 mL/100 mL blood/mmHg at 37°C, then the amount of O_2 removed is calculated as follows:

   $60 \times 0.003 = 0.18$ mL

2. *Use this figure to calculate the amount of O_2 carried by plasma.* If a total of 5 mL of O_2 per 100 mL of blood is being used and 0.18 mL of this is coming from plasma, then the amount of O_2 being used at a tissue level, i.e., being carried by the plasma, is calculated as follows:

   $0.18/5 \times 100 = 3.6\%$

Note: Henry's law (see Appendix 2) states that the quantity of gas dissolved in a liquid at a given temperature is directly proportional to the partial pressure of the gas to which the liquid is exposed. This, of course, does not take into account chemical reactions. The solubility coefficient for O_2 is 0.003 mL/100 mL of blood/mmHg at 37°C. Units per mmHg are easier to use for our purposes.

If 3.6% of the O_2 is being carried in the plasma, then 96.4% is being carried in some other way. The RBC is responsible for carrying the remainder of O_2.

Oxygen Carried by the RBC

The vast majority of O_2 transported in the blood is combined with hemoglobin contained in the RBC. Normal values for males are 14.0–18.0 g/dL and for

TABLE 9-1 Normal Values for Hemoglobin		
	g/dL	g/L
Males	14.0–18.0	140–180
Females	12.0–16.0	120–160
Newborns	13.5–21.5	135–215
One-year-olds	11.0–13.5	110–135
Ten-year-olds	11.5–15.0	115–150

females 12–16 g/dL (Table 9-1). In females, lower levels of 2,3-diphosphoglycerate (DPG) in RBCs allow for a more efficient carrying of O_2, which preserves the efficiency of these lower hemoglobin levels. It is the unique physiological ability of hemoglobin to combine reversibly with O_2 that gives the RBC its ability to carry large quantities of O_2. When full, each gram of hemoglobin can carry 1.34 mL of O_2 (the theoretical maximum is 1.39 mL, but for our purposes 1.34 mL will be used).

Reversible Combination (Affinity)

O_2 must combine with hemoglobin in the lungs and then be released when it arrives in the tissues. The ability of hemoglobin to pick up O_2 is termed affinity. Hemoglobin's affinity for O_2 is said to increase anywhere in the lung where the need exists to pick up O_2. Decreased affinity means hemoglobin's ability to combine with O_2 is reduced. This occurs at the tissue level, where O_2 must be released for use.

The oxyhemoglobin dissociation curve describes the ability of hemoglobin to combine with O_2 under various physiological conditions. Figure 9-1 represents the relationship between the blood partial pressure of O_2 and how full the hemoglobin is (expressed as a percentage and commonly referred to as saturation).

P_{50} describes the partial pressure at which the hemoglobin is 50% saturated, or full of O_2. A decreased P_{50} indicates that 50% saturation occurs at a lower PO_2 and an increased P_{50} indicates that 50% saturation occurs at a higher PO_2.

The sigmoid shape of the oxyhemoglobin dissociation curve occurs as a result of changing affinities of hemoglobin for O_2. These changes are a result of the heme–heme interaction sometimes referred to as the molecular lung, a condition that is identified by the actual movement of heme into and out of the molecule.

Increased Affinity

When blood enters the lung from the right side of the heart (mixed venous blood), the affinity of hemoglobin for O_2 increases. This facilitates the uptake of O_2, which is desirable for the necessary rapid absorption of O_2 into the blood from the lungs (Figure 9-2).

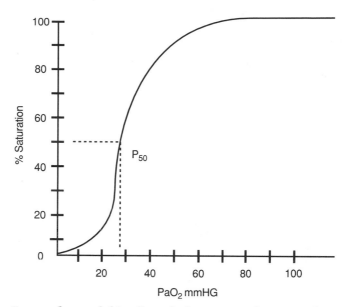

Figure 9-1.   Oxygen-hemoglobin dissociation curve. The normal curve bisects the point where O_2 saturation is 50% and PaO_2 is 27 mm of mercury.

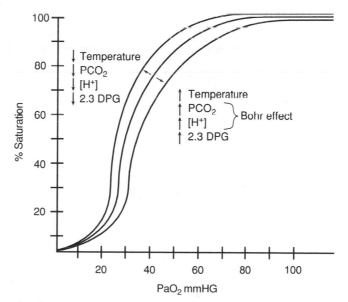

Figure 9-2.   The four primary factors that cause a shift of the oxyhemoglobin dissociation curves and change the affinity of hemoglobin for oxygen.

TABLE 9-2 Normal Blood Gas Values		
	Arterial	Mixed Venous*
Oxygen Content (mL/dL)	20	15
Saturation	98%	75%
CO_2 Content (mL/dL)	49	53
pH	7.40	7.30

* This pulmonary artery sample is referred to as mixed because it is a mixture of blood from all regions of the body.

The Bohr effect describes the increased affinity seen as blood enters the lung. When blood enters the right side of the heart it is low in O_2 content, high in CO_2 content, and has a low pH (Table 9-2).

Alveolar ventilation reduces CO_2 and increases pH, resulting in a shift of the oxyhemoglobin dissociation curve to the left (Figure 9-3). This improves hemoglobin's ability to pick up O_2. This saturation of the blood with O_2 also facilitates the release of CO_2. The effect that O_2 saturation has on hemoglobin's ability to carry CO_2 is referred to as the Haldane effect (see next page for full details).

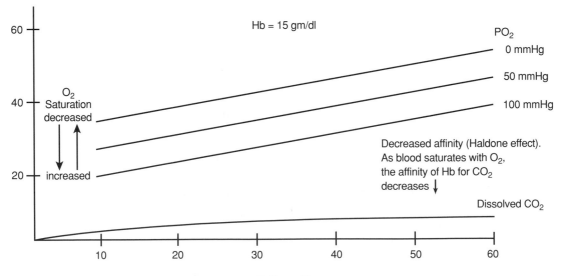

Figure 9-3. The dissociation of carbon dioxide from hemoglobin also can be represented by a dissociation curve. The relationship between the content of carbon dioxide in plasma and the partial pressure of carbon dioxide is not a linear relationship.

A decrease in 2,3-DPG and a decrease in body temperature also cause an increase in the affinity of hemoglobin for O_2. An increase in 2,3-DPG and an increase in body temperature also shifts the curve to the right, decreasing the affinity of hemoglobin for O_2.

Decreased Affinity

When blood enters the tissues after leaving the left side of the heart (arterial blood), the affinity of hemoglobin for O_2 decreases (Figure 9-3). This facilitates the rapid release of O_2, a desirable feature that enhances the speedy oxygenation of tissues. The **Bohr effect** also describes the decrease in affinity of hemoglobin for O_2, seen as blood enters the tissue capillary bed. The arterial blood is relatively high in O_2, low in CO_2, and high in pH. The production of CO_2 by normal aerobic metabolism decreases pH and increases CO_2 levels. This impacts on the oxyhemoglobin dissociation curve by shifting it to the right.

This shift reflects the release of O_2 into the tissues for use. This desaturation of the hemoglobin increases its ability to carry CO_2. This phenomenon is also referred to as the **Haldane effect**.

Oxygen Cascade

The **oxygen cascade** describes the decrease in O_2 partial pressure seen as O_2 travels from ambient air into the lungs and out to the tissues via the arterial blood.

▼ CARBON DIOXIDE TRANSPORT

CO_2 transport through the bloodstream is achieved via three different mechanisms. Some portion of CO_2 is (1) dissolved in the plasma, and the remainder is either (2) transported as carbaminohemoglobin or (3) ferried via the bicarbonate mechanism.

Approximately 4 mL of CO_2 is absorbed and released from every 100 mL of blood per minute. Therefore, arterial PCO_2 is approximately 49 mL/dL and mixed venous blood is approximately 53 mL/dL. The majority of CO_2, approximately 60–70%, is carried via the bicarbonate mechanism; approximately 20–25% is carried as carbaminohemoglobin; 5–10% is carried as dissolved CO_2 in the plasma.

Carbon Dioxide Dissolved in Plasma

CO_2 is the product of normal aerobic metabolism. Its continuous production creates a pressure gradient out of the cells and into the blood. As CO_2 enters the blood it dissolves in the plasma. Its solubility coefficient is 0.067 mL/dL/mmHg/37°C. Even with this high solubility coefficient, only 5–10% of the CO_2 is carried in this form. Even though very little CO_2 is dissolved in plasma, this mechanism is essential to the transport of CO_2 across the plasma medium and into the RBCs. A small amount of CO_2 in plasma also combines with water to form carbonic acid (H_2CO_3), which dissociates to produce bicarbonate ions (HCO_3^-) and hydrogen ions (H^+):

$$CO_2 + H_2O \rightarrow H_2CO_3 \; H^+ + HCO_3^-$$

This reaction occurs very slowly in plasma, making it insignificant to the transport of CO_2.

Carbaminohemoglobin

Between 20% and 30% of the CO_2 is carried in combination with plasma proteins and by hemoglobin inside the RBC. Plasma proteins account for about 25% of this mechanism; the remaining 75% results from the combination with hemoglobin inside the RBC. This combination is a loss bond, easily reversed by a pressure gradient once inside the lung.

Bicarbonate Mechanism

The RBC contains an enzyme known as carbonic anhydrase. This enzyme catalyzes (speeds up) the reaction between CO_2 and water, thus facilitating the production of H^+ and HCO_3^-. Once dissociated, the H^+ combines with the hemoglobin molecule, and HCO_3^- diffuses outside the cell into the plasma. Chloride diffuses from the plasma into the RBC to maintain chemical neutral-

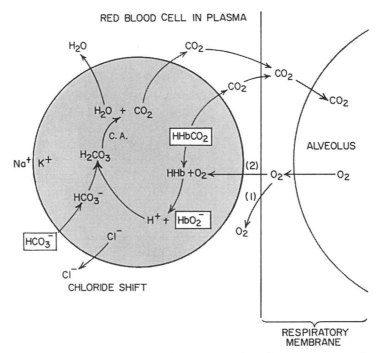

Figure 9-4.   The shift in ions. (Chaffee, E.E. and Lytle, I.M., Basic Physiology and Anatomy, 4th ed. Philadelphia: J.B. Lippincott, 1980, with permission.)

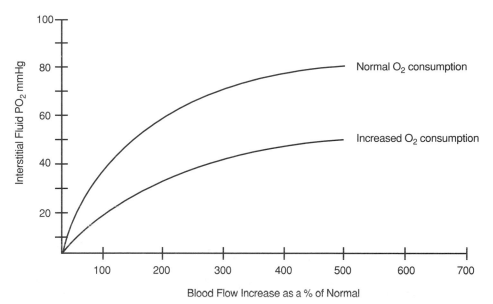

Figure 9-5.   The rate of capillary flow impacts on interstitial fluid PO_2. As blood flows through the capillary bed of a particular tissue, greater quantities of oxygen are transported into the tissue in a given period of time. The opposite occurs as tissue perfusion decreases.

ity. This transfer of ions is known as the chloride shift, or **Hamburger phenomenon** (Figure 9-4). Specialized carrier molecules in the RBC membrane make this transport of ions rapid.

The shift in ions results in a water influx into the RBC and an outflow of water that occurs when the RBC arrives in the lung (Figure 9-4). This process is completely reversible when the RBCs enter the pulmonary capillary bed. The entire process responds to a pressure gradient (Figures 9.5 and 9.6). In the tissues, where CO_2 is being produced, CO_2 moves into the RBC with H^+ combining with hemoglobin and HCO_3^- diffusing out into the plasma. When this blood reaches the pulmonary capillary bed, bicarbonate returns inside the RBC, combines with H^+, and forms carbonic acid, which dissociates into CO_2 and water. The water diffuses outside the cell again and CO_2 diffuses into the plasma, then out into the alveoli, where it is eventually exhaled out of the lungs (Figure 9-4).

▼ THE HEMOGLOBIN MOLECULE

When protein is attached to an iron-containing pigment, it is referred to as **conjugated protein**. The conjugated protein hemoglobin is made up of an iron-containing porphyrin ring called *heme* and a water-soluble protein called *globin*.

The uniqueness of this molecule lies in its ability to reversibly bind with O_2. Even small changes in the structure of the hemoglobin molecule can result

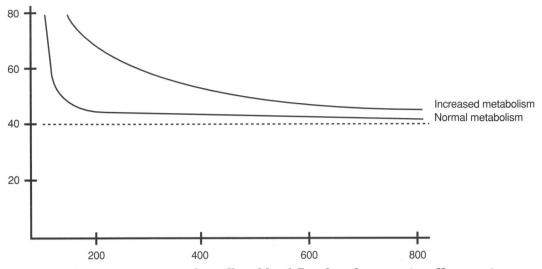

Figure 9-6. Increased capillary blood flow has the opposite effect on tissue PCO₂ as it has on O₂. As blood flow decreases into the capillaries of a particular tissue, PCO₂ increases.

in impairment of its ability to carry O_2. Hemoglobin has a molecular weight of 64,458, which is an indication of just how complex the molecule is.

Heme

Heme is an iron-centered molecule with four pyrrol groups linked by methene bridges. Combined, the pyrrol groups are referred to as a porphyrin molecule. There are four heme groups per hemoglobin molecule, each of which can carry one O_2 molecule. Therefore, each hemoglobin molecule can carry four O_2 molecules (eight atoms) (Figure 9-7).

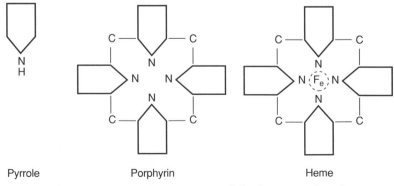

Figure 9-7. Basic structure of the heme molecule.

The heme molecule normally exists in its ferrous state, in which case it is referred to as **methemoglobin**, discussed later in this chapter (see "Methemoglobin"). To carry O_2, it must remain in its reduced state. Oxidation to its ferrous state renders it incapable of carrying O_2. (Although it is not chemically correct, *reduced hemoglobin* is a more commonly used term referring to hemoglobin without O_2.)

Globin

Globin is the protein portion of the hemoglobin molecule. The sequence of amino acids in these polypeptide chains (protein) results in their differentia-

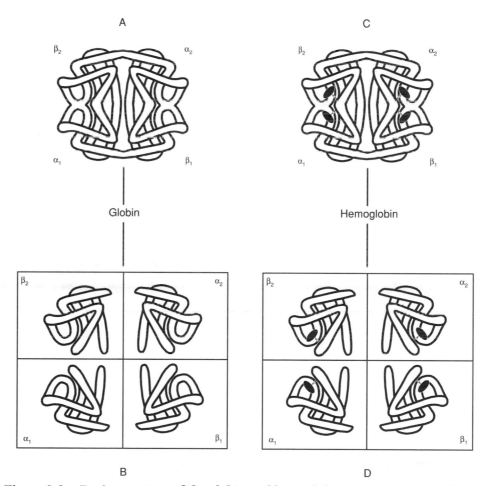

Figure 9-8. **Basic structure of the globin and hemoglobin molecules. Note that the ferrous ion FE^{+6} has four sites combined with the pyrrol groups, one site combined with the globin chain, and only one site remains to combine with oxygen. (Adapted from: Henry, J.B., Clinical Diagnosis and Management by Laboratory Methods, 17th ed. Philadelphia: W.B. Saunders, 1984, with permission.)**

tion. Researchers can identify variations in the structure or sequence of these polypeptide chains, designated alpha (α), beta (β), gamma (γ), and delta (Δ) For a graphic representation of the heme and globin (hemoglobin), see Figure 9-8.

Hemoglobin A, adult hemoglobin, contains two α and two β chains. The α chain contains 141 amino acids and the β chain contains 146 amino acids. **Hemoglobin F**, or fetal hemoglobin, has two α and two γ chains. **Hemoglobin A$_2$** is a variation of adult hemoglobin that has two α chains and two Δ chains.

Globin is the portion of the hemoglobin molecule responsible for combining with the H^+ and CO_2. This enables the molecule to act as a buffer for acid–base balance. (See Chapter 13 for an expanded discussion of acid–base balance.)

▼ ABNORMALITIES IN GAS TRANSPORT

Lack of sufficient hemoglobin (anemia) can significantly reduce O_2-carrying capacity, and excessive RBC concentration (polycythemia) can result in impeded blood flow because the blood thickens (increasing viscosity).

RBC production is stimulated by anything that affects O_2 delivery to the tissues. Anemia, high altitude, lung disease, and heart failure all can stimulate an increase in the production of RBCs. The primary factor responsible for this increased production is the hormone erythropoietin. Hypoxia results in an increase in production of erythropoietin in the kidney. Without erythropoietin, hypoxia has little or no effect on RBC production.

The transport of gases between the tissues and the lungs can be significantly affected by a number of abnormalities. Impeded transport may result from one of any number of factors:

1. Reduced blood flow
2. Anemia
3. Hemoglobinopathies
4. Thalassemia
5. Cyanide poisoning
6. Carboxyhemoglobin
7. Methemoglobin
8. Sulfhemoglobin

Reduced Blood Flow

Gas transport is dependent on two factors: (1) the amount of gas carried in a given volume of blood and (2) the quantity and/or availability of circulating blood. Reduced blood flow to the entire body, or a part thereof, results in a reduction of the gases transported. The affected regions have a resulting hypoxia and acidosis. This hypoxia, seen when there is insufficient blood supply, is commonly referred to as **circulatory hypoxia** or **stagnant hypoxia** (Figure 9-6).

Anemia

Anemia is a term used to describe a deficiency of RBCs. In broad terms, this deficiency is attributed to one of two conditions: rapid loss (bleeding) or inadequate production. When RBCs are not present in the blood in sufficient quantities, gas transport is severely hindered. Remember, the amount of O_2 carried in the blood is dependent on the number of grams of hemoglobin carried in the RBCs.

Anemia may be a result of

1. rapid blood loss.
2. aplastic anemia.
3. megaloblastic anemia.
4. hemolytic anemia.

Rapid Blood Loss

Hemorrhage (another way of referring to rapid blood loss) results in a reduced RBC concentration. This is because it takes the body 20–30 days to replace the RBCs lost, although it can replace the lost plasma within 24–72 hours. If the blood loss continues for a long enough period of time, the body may not be able to keep up with the iron loss. This results in RBCs being produced with insufficient hemoglobin inside, a condition known as **microcytic hypochromic anemia**.

Aplastic Anemia

This rare anemia is expressed as a lack of RBCs resulting from insufficiently functioning bone marrow. This may be a result of radiation or chemical poisoning.

Megaloblastic Anemia

Megaloblastic anemia results from a deficiency in one of the factors responsible for the production of *erythroblasts* (immature erythrocytes) in the bone marrow. The resulting slow reproduction produces large, oddly shaped cells known as *megaloblasts*. These cells are not produced in sufficient quantities for gas transport.

Hemolytic Anemia

A common result of a hereditary disorder, hemolytic anemia is characterized by fragile RBCs that rupture easily. This RBC destruction (**hemolysis**) results in an insufficient number of cells available for gas transport.

Hemoglobinopathies

A **hemoglobinopathy** is any abnormality in hemoglobin structure that can lead to accelerated RBC destruction (**hemolytic anemia**). The two major types of hemoglobinopathies that can result in RBC hemolysis are sickle cell anemia and thalassemia.

Sickle Cell Anemia

This disease is defined by the abnormal substitution of an amino acid in the hemoglobin molecule. This is the most commonly encountered hemoglobinopathy.

Thalassemia

This group of hereditary disorders results in a defect in the synthesis of one or more of the polypeptide chains of hemoglobin. This defect is expressed as either a failure of or a decrease in the synthesis of the affected chain. The RBCs are small (microcytic) and contain a low content of hemoglobin (hypochromic).

α **Thalassemia** is characterized by impaired synthesis of the α chain. β **Thalassemia** is expressed as a reduction or absence of the β chains. The effect on gas transport can be significant in those with the homozygous form of beta chain synthesis deficiency (thalassemia major), but it is usually mild for those who are heterozygous for either α or β chain synthesis deficiency.

Cyanide Poisoning

This is a classic example of the tissue's inability to use O_2 as the direct result of the complete blockage of the action of cytochrome oxidase. This enzyme is important to biological oxidation because it transfers electrons from cytochrome for use of O_2. Cytochrome oxidase effectively activates O_2 to unite with hydrogen to form water in the Kreb cycle.

When the action of cytochrome oxidase is blocked, O_2 transport remains completely normal but the tissues become incapable of using O_2. As a result, hypoxia exists even in the presence of high concentrations of O_2.

Carboxyhemoglobin

Carbon monoxide is an odorless, colorless, poisonous gas that is found in exhaust and smoking tobacco, among other sources. It combines with hemoglobin at the same position normally occupied by O_2. This reduces hemoglobin's O_2 transport capabilities to a significant degree because hemoglobin has an affinity for carbon monoxide over 200 times greater than its affinity for O_2.

With a partial pressure of less than 0.5 mmHg, carbon monoxide will compete one on one with O_2's partial pressure of 100 mmHg. A carbon monoxide pressure of 0.7 mmHg can be lethal because it can reduce O_2-carrying capacity to a level incompatible with life.

The symptoms of carbon monoxide poisoning are variable (racing heart, dizziness, muscle weakness, nausea, ringing in the ear), but typically include deep, difficult respiration. This condition is treated by removing the source of carbon monoxide and administering 100% O_2 under hyperbaric pressure (1.5–3 times atmospheric pressure).

Methemoglobin

When the iron of the hemoglobin molecule assumes the ferric form by losing an electron, it is referred to as methemoglobin. In this state it is incapable of carrying O_2. This can occur whenever reducing agents, such as ascorbic acid and methylene blue, are present in the bloodstream. Patients with methemoglobinemia have a deficiency of the necessary enzymes responsible for converting methemoglobin back to hemoglobin.

Sulfhemoglobin

This compound, also called sulmethemoglobin, results when hemoglobin combines with hydrogen sulfide. When this occurs, hemoglobin cannot carry O_2. A number of drugs with hydrogen sulfide can produce this condition.

▼ CONCLUSION

Gas transport from the lungs into the tissues and back to the lungs is essential for life. This chapter has described both O_2 and CO_2 transport. With the basics presented here in hand, readers should be able to move on to the real challenge of acquainting themselves with the heart and systemic circulation.

❖ Review Questions

1. Oxygen is carried primarily by/in
   a. plasma.
   b. serum.
   c. hemoglobin.
   d. globin.
   e. myoglobin.
2. The solubility coefficient of oxygen is
   a. 0.003 mL/dL/mmHg at 37°C.
   b. 0.03 mL/dL at 37°C.
   c. 0.067 mL/dL/mmHg at 37°C.
   d. 0.3 mL/dL/mmHg at 37°C
   e. 1.2 mL/dL/mmHg at 37°C.
3. The quantity of gas dissolved in a liquid at a given temperature is directly proportional to the partial pressure of the gas to which the liquid is exposed. This is ____ law.
   a. Graham's
   b. Boyle's
   c. Starling's

    d. Henry's

    e. Haldane's

4. The mean values for arterial oxygen content, mL/dL saturation (%), and pH are
    a. 15, 75, and 7.36.
    b. 21, 80, and 7.45.
    c. 25, 810, and 7.5.
    d. 20, 108, and 7.4.
    e. 26, 100, and 7.35.

5. Which of the factors shifts the oxyhemoglobin dissociation curve to the right?
    i. Increased temperature
    ii. Increased hydrogen in concentration
    iii. Decreased pH.
    iv. Decreased PCO_2
    v. Increased 2,3-DPG

    a. i, ii, iii
    b. ii, iii, iv
    c. iii, iv, v
    d. i, ii, iii, iv, v
    e. All of the above

6. As blood saturates with O_2, the decreasing affinity of Hb for CO_2 is known as _____ law.
    a. Haldane's
    b. Graham's
    c. Boyle's
    d. Charles'
    e. Bohr's

7. Carbon dioxide is carried in the blood
    i. dissolved in the plasma.
    ii. as myoglobin.
    iii. as carbaminohemoglobin.
    iv. by cytochrome P_{450}.
    v. through the bicarbonate mechanism.

    a. i, ii, iii
    b. ii, iii, iv
    c. i, iii, v
    d. iii, iv, v
    e. i, ii, iii

8. Hemoglobin A consists of
    i. two alpha chains.
    ii. two gamma chains.
    iii. two delta chains.
    iv. two beta chains.
    v. two theta chains.

    a. i, iv
    b. i, v
    c. ii, iv
    d. iii, iv
    e. ii, iii

9. Normal male hemoglobin is (g/L)
    a. 60–80.
    b. 80–100.
    c. 140–180.
    d. 150–170.
    e. 180–200.

10. Red blood cells function for approximately _____ days.
    a. 20
    b. 30
    c. 60
    d. 80
    e. 120

10

THE HEART

OBJECTIVES

1. Review the anatomy of the heart.

2. Describe the basic physiology of heart muscle.

3. Detail the process of synchronization of cardiac muscle.

4. Explain the concept of action potential.

5. List the four phases of cardiac muscle contraction.

6. Describe myocardial contraction in terms of the sliding filament model.

7. Outline the steps in a single cardiac cycle.

Matthews LR: CARDIOPULMONARY ANATOMY AND PHYSIOLOGY. © 1996 Lippincott–Raven Publishers.

8. Characterize the fundamental heart sounds.

9. Describe the electrocardiogram in terms of depolarization, repolarization, and generation of the ECG.

10. Account for myocardial performance in terms of preload, afterload, contractility, and heart rate.

11. Enumerate the ventricular functions.

12. Determine the impact of mechanical ventilation on cardiac output.

13. Describe the neuronal control over cardiac function.

14. Describe the impact electrolytes have on myocardial function.

15. Review the anatomy of coronary blood flow.

16. Enumerate the basic cardiac dysrhythmias.

The heart, a hollow, muscular organ that lies at the center of the circulatory system, provides the force for circulating blood throughout the vascular system. Its central role in routing circulation makes it the ideal point of departure for discussing the cardiovascular network's implication in cardiopulmonary functioning. (The circulatory system proper is addressed in Chapter 11.)

This dynamic organ is enclosed in a fibroserous membrane called the *pericardial sac* and consists of two separate pumps: the right side and the left side. The right side receives blood from the body via the inferior and superior venae cavae and pumps it into the lungs via the pulmonary arteries. The left side receives blood from the lungs via the pulmonary veins and pumps it out into the entire body (initially via the aorta). Pulmonary circulation is covered in depth in its own chapter (see Chapter 7), rather than as part of the chapter on systemic circulation, to emphasize the importance of its contribution to ventilation.

Each side of the heart contains an *atrium* and a *ventricle* (Figure 10-1). Although the atrium is capable of pumping, its action is weak and its primary function is to service a ventricle by assisting in filling it with blood. The ventricle provides the primary force that sends blood out into the lungs and the rest of the body. This chapter describes the heart's function as a pump and the mechanisms of its regulation.

Figures 10-1 and 10-2, which provide useful orienting views of both the exterior and interior of the heart, are a fitting introduction to basic heart muscle physiology.

▼ BASIC HEART MUSCLE PHYSIOLOGY

The heart wall contains three distinct layers: the *epicardium* (the outer serous layer), the *endocardium* (the inner layer that lines the four chambers of the

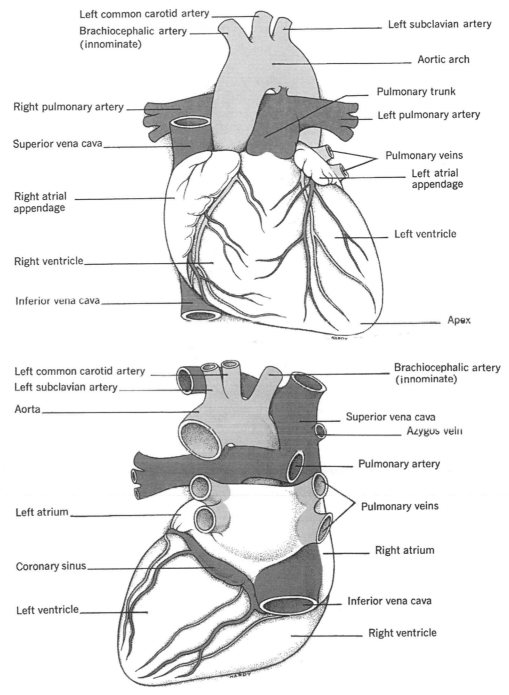

Figure 10-1.   Anatomy of the heart. (Chaffee, E.E. and Lytle, I.M., Basic Physiology and Anatomy, 4th ed. Philadelphia: J.B. Lippincott, 1980, with permission.)

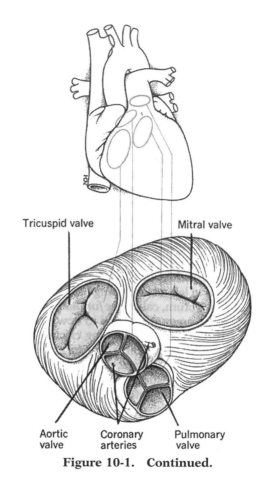

Figure 10-1.   Continued.

heart and its valves), and, sandwiched between them, the *myocardium*. The myocardium is invested with three types of muscle:

1. Atrial muscle. This muscle, which is thinner and less complicated than ventricular muscle, has a short refractory period. The short rest period between contractions affords this muscle the power to achieve a higher rate of contraction.
2. Ventricular muscle. This muscle is a comparatively more complex fiber than atrial muscle. It also has a shorter refractory period.
3. Specialized muscle. This muscle consists of excitatory and conductive fibers. These muscles, which contain few contractile fibers, are capable of weak contraction. However, their ability to conduct rapidly makes these fibers the ideal vehicle for conveying a network of excitatory and conductive impulses throughout the heart.

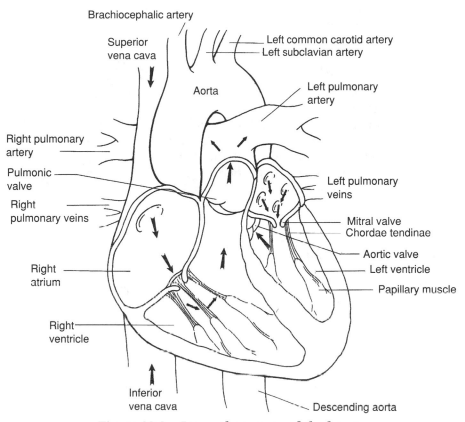

Figure 10 2.   Internal anatomy of the heart.

The myocardium is important because it is an arrangement of cylindrically shaped striated muscle fibers 10–15 μm wide and 30–60 μm long. These muscles function in the same way that muscle fibers function anywhere else in the body.

In short, depolarization of the sarcolemma generates an electrical potential that travels along the *transverse tubules* (t-tubules) to the interior of the cell, where it causes depolarization of the *cisternal membranes* of the sarcoplasmic reticulum. T-tubules are a channel-like system that connects the sarcolemma and extends into the myocardial fiber. These tubules are filled with interstitial fluid and run along the myocardial cells. Depolarization of the sarcolemma generates an electrical potential that travels along the t-tubules to the interior of the cell, where it causes depolarization of the cisternal membranes of the sarcoplasmic reticulum. The cisternae release calcium ions, which activate myosin to split adenosine triphosphate (ATP). The resulting energy release allows for the formation of cross-bridges between actin and myosin, causing contraction of the muscle. The sarcoplasmic reticulum then again takes up calcium and returns the sarcomere to a relaxed state. (See Chapter 1 for a review of muscle physiology.)

▼ SYNCHRONIZATION OF THE CARDIAC MUSCLE

Cardiac muscle is, in actuality, a network of individual cardiac muscle cells. The membrane between these cells is permeable to ion transfers, resulting in a syncytium, or mass of protoplasm, that makes the system function almost as a single cell. This occurs in the atrium and the ventricles. However, a fibrous tissue layer separates the two regions, which results in a time lag between contractions of the atrium and ventricle. This is important for the normal function of the heart.

▼ ACTION POTENTIAL

Normal cardiac muscle has a resting membrane potential of approximately -90 mV. This means that the difference in electrical charge between the inside and the outside of the cell at rest creates an electrical pressure gradient of -90 mV. The resting membrane potential is significant because it is an indication of the cell's potential for a given amount of work.

The action potential, which arises in response to nerve or muscle fiber stimulation, increases to $+20$ mV during contraction. This contraction is referred to as depolarization. The membrane remains in this depolarized state for approximately 0.2 seconds for atrial muscle and 0.3 seconds for ventricular muscle. This creates a plateau (or refractory period) before the cell begins to repolarize. The purpose of this plateau is to promote efficient, forceful myocardial contractions by maintaining appropriate levels of calcium and potassium ions within the cell (Figure 10-3).

Contraction of the cardiac muscle is a result of an ion influx into the muscle fiber. Two channels exist: (1) the fast channel for sodium (Na^+) ions and (2) the slow channel for calcium (Ca^{+2}) and Na^+ ions. The first process creates the necessary immediate response but not the following plateau. The second process occurs slowly, keeping the muscle in a depolarized state. The calcium that enters the cell is important for the force of contraction of the muscle cell. The presence of calcium in the cell also reduces the outflux of potassium (K^+), further preventing recovery of the cell to its precontraction state.

The cyclical nature of the phases of the action potential allow the cells to exist in a state of readiness:

1. Phase 0 represents a rapid depolarization, which is caused by direct stimulation of the muscle or, in the case of myocardial muscle, orchestrated by internal pacemakers (see "The Sinoatrial Node"). This action potential is initiated by a dramatic increase

Systole

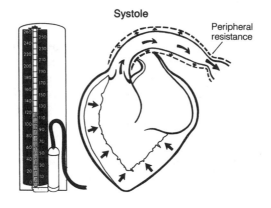

Peripheral resistance

Diastole

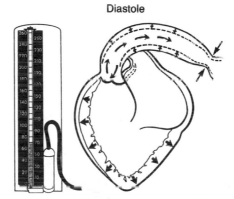

Figure 10-3.   Diagram showing direction of blood flow during diastole and systole. (Porth, C.M., Pathophysiology: Concepts of Altered Health States, 4th ed. Philadelphia: J.B. Lippincott, 1994, with permission.)

in Na^+ membrane permeability. The Na^+ rushes through the ion-specific channels (fast channels), rapidly creating a positive voltage, which prompts muscle cell contraction.

2. Phase 1 corresponds to an absolute refractory period, during which further contraction of the cell is impossible, regardless of the amount of stimulation applied. The increased Na^+ permeability is rapidly inactivated as the cell begins repolarization.

3. Phase 2 is characterized by a delay in repolarization caused by an increased permeability of Ca^{+2} through the ion-specific channels (slow channels). The influx of Ca^{+2} maintains voltage potential at 10 to -20 mV for over 100 msec.

4. Phase 3 represents a rapid move toward complete repolarization. This is a result of inactivation of the Ca^{+2} permeability and an increase in K^+ permeability.

5. Phase 4, which actually serves as the end point for the previous

action potential, represents resting membrane potential with normal concentration gradients for K^+ and Na^+ ions maintained by active ion pumping as well as by selective membrane permeability to these ions. During phase 4, the spontaneous diastolic depolarization of a muscle cell occurs. This slow depolarization is characteristic of pacemaker cells in the heart. When the threshold potential is reached (usually at -60 mV), Na^+ permeability is again dramatically increased and phase 0 begins again.

During the refractory period (phase 1) the muscle cannot be stimulated, and during the relative refractory period (phase 2) the muscle cell is difficult to stimulate. This refractory phase is extremely important in stabilizing the myocardium. An increase in the refractory period results in the heart's inability to respond to frequent stimulation and also decreases myocardial irritability. A decrease in the refractory period can result in the muscle cell's increased ability to respond as well as to an increase in myocardial irritability.

Remember that the atria have a shorter refractory period than the ventricles. This means that the contraction rate of the atria can be much faster than that of the ventricles.

▼ MYOCARDIAL CONTRACTION

The strength of the myocardial contraction is dependent on the concentration of extracellular calcium ions. Calcium ion concentrations in both the t-tubule system and the extracellular fluid have an impact on cardiac contractile strength. Contraction of the myocardium begins milliseconds after the action potential begins and ends milliseconds after it stops. The length of time for an action potential, and therefore a contraction, is decreased as heart rate (HR) is increased. Normally, the contraction phase (systole) of the cardiac cycle is approximately 40% of the total cardiac cycle. This leaves 60% of the cycle for the ventricle to refill (diastole).

When HR is increased, the contraction phase begins to take up more of the cardiac cycle. If the HR is increased too much (tachycardia), the ventricles may not have time to refill before the next contraction. This can potentially reduce cardiac output to a dangerous level.

Sliding Filament Model

The tension developed by the cardiac muscle is proportional to the number of cross-bridges between the actin and myosin myofilaments. The greater the number of force-generating sites, the stronger the contraction. The number of sites is increased as the sarcomere increases in length to a maximum of 2.2 μm. This fundamental property of cardiac muscle gives it the ability to increase its force of contraction as it is stretched (Starling's law of heart*).

---

* Starling's law of heart states that the heartbeat is determined primarily by the length of the fibers in its muscular wall.

▼ THE CARDIAC CYCLE

The cardiac cycle describes the period of time from the beginning of one contraction to the beginning of the next. It consists of a period of contraction (systole) followed by a period of relaxation (diastole). This cycle results in blood pressure changes and hence blood volume movement. These changes are referred to as **hemodynamics**. (See Figure 10-3 for a depiction of the direction of blood flow during ventricular diastole and systole.)

Figure 10-4 represents the hemodynamic events that occur during the course of a normal cardiac cycle. During the diastolic period, the ventricles fill with blood. The P wave of the electrocardiogram (ECG) shows the electrical excitation of the atrium (Figure 10-4). As the electrical impulse spreads over the atrium, the atrial muscle contracts to cause an increase in both atrial and ventricular pressures. The opening of the *mitral valve* (between the left atrium and left ventricle) and the *tricuspid valve* (between the right atrium and right ventricle) allows for the transmission of this pressure to the ventricles (Figure

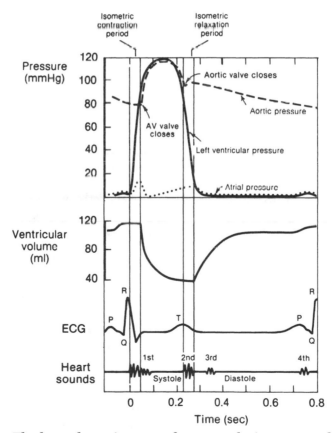

Figure 10-4. The hemodynamic events that occur during a normal cardiac cycle. (Porth, C.M., Pathophysiology: Concepts of Altered Health States, 4th ed. Philadelphia: J.B. Lippincott, 1994, with permission.)

10-2). Approximately 80% of the ventricular filling occurs during diastole, so atrial contraction contributes only a small amount to ventricular volume.

As the electrical stimulus moves into the ventricles via the atrioventricular (A-V) node, bundle of His, and the Purkinje fibers (all of which are described in the section "The Electrocardiogram"), ventricular contraction occurs. Ventricular depolarization is characterized by the QRS complex of the ECG. (The QRS complex is a graphic representation of the path of an excitatory wave through the heart. The Q wave corresponds to the initial downward deflection, the R to a large upward deflection, and the S to the spread of the electrical impulse from the Purkinje fibers to the ventricular muscle.)

When the ventricles contract, intraventricular pressure begins to increase. The A-V valves (mitral and tricuspid valves) close, creating the first heart sound (the "lubb" of the classic "lubb-dubb"). When the ventricles first contract and pressure begins to increase, the A-V valves are closed, as are the pulmonic and aortic valves. Initially, this means that blood is not exiting the ventricle. Because the blood is not compressible, pressure increases rapidly, making this time period short (less than 50 msec). No blood moves during this period, which is why it is termed the isovolumic phase of contraction.

As the pressure increases, it exceeds the pressure in the pulmonary artery and the aorta. When this happens, the pulmonic and aortic valves open and systole begins. Ejection of blood is quick at first and then decreases throughout systole. During rest, when the HR is approximately 72 beats/min, systole lasts for approximately 0.3 seconds. Once the ventricle has contracted, relaxation begins and the pressure decreases. At this point both the pulmonic and aortic valves close, causing the second heart sound.

When the aortic valve closes, it causes a sharp notch in arterial pressure. The notch created by this pressure change is known as the **dicrotic notch**. The notch is caused by blood temporarily flowing back into the left ventricle just before closure of the aortic valve. When the valve closes, the backflow stops abruptly and pressure increases briefly, causing a notch. The notch is followed by a gradual decrease in pressure, back to the diastolic pressure level. Blood continues to flow even during diastole because the elastic recoil of the arterial walls maintains a pressure gradient. Ventricular repolarization is characterized by the T wave of the ECG (caused by repolarization of the ventricles).

When ventricular pressure decreases below atrial pressure, the A-V valves open and the ventricles begin to fill rapidly. As the blood flows into the ventricle, atrial pressure decreases but flow is maintained by a corresponding decrease in ventricular pressure due to ventricular relaxation. This rapid filling time lasts little more than 100 msec, and for the remainder of diastole the ventricles fill by venous return pressures alone.

Venous pulsation has been recorded in the major veins. Three positive waves have been recorded: a, c, and v wave forms. The a wave results from the contraction of the right atrium. The c wave results from the closure of the tricuspid valve at the beginning of ventricular contraction. The v wave results from the gradual increase in pressure from venous return during systole.

▼ HEART SOUNDS

There are essentially four heart sounds, although generally only the first two are audible with a stethoscope. The first heart sound ("lubb") is heard during auscultation. This "lubb" is a result of A-V valve closure, blood ejecting out of the aortic opening, and the myocardial contraction.

The second heart sound ("dubb") is caused by closure of the aortic and pulmonic valves. The third sound is believed to result from the rapid filling of the ventricles and is rarely audible in adults. Exercise and certain pathologic states may produce this sound. The fourth sound results from contraction of the atrium but is generally not audible with a stethoscope.

▼ THE ELECTROCARDIOGRAM

The ECG is a recording of the electrical voltages generated by the heart, not pump function. It is an effective diagnostic tool for identifying abnormal cardiac rhythms and pathologic states. However, a sound understanding of the normal ECG must be present before abnormalities can be addressed. In Figure 10-5, the relationship between the ECG and the cardiac cycle is represented. Remember that the ECG does not represent pump function.

Heart Depolarization

Depolarization of the myocardium results in a negative charge in relationship to other polarized regions. The electrical current flows from the positively

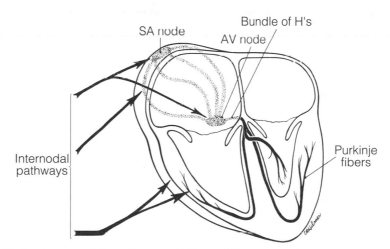

Figure 10-5.   Internodal pathways. (Adapted from: Porth, C.M., Pathophysiology: Concepts of Altered Health States, 4th ed. Philadelphia: J.B. Lippincott, 1994, with permission.)

charged portion of the myocardium, through the conductive medium, toward the negatively charged region of the myocardium, creating muscle contraction along the way. The electrical charge developed by depolarization and repolarization of the heart sets up a two-pole (dipole) environment that can be measured by specialized equipment. Two electrodes placed inside this electrical environment can record variation in the electrical field based on

1. the magnitude of the voltage.
2. the position of the electrodes with respect to the direction of depolarization.
3. the distance of the electrodes from the generated electrical charge.

Generating the ECG

The adult heart contracts at a rate of approximately 72 beats/min. Figure 10-5 illustrates the specialized conduction network responsible for the rhythmic and controlled cardiac contractions.

The electrical impulse normally originates in the sinoatrial (S-A) node. It then travels out and down the internodal pathways to the A-V node, through the bundle of His, and into the right and left bundle branches. Finally, impulses spread out into the Purkinje fibers (muscle fibers that lie under the endocardium and form the electrical impulse conducting system), where the impulse contacts all parts of the ventricles.

The Sinoatrial Node: Origin of the P Wave

The S-A node is an area of specialized muscle tissue approximately 3 mm wide, 15 mm long, and 1 mm thick. It is located in the wall of the right atrium near the entrance to the superior *vena cava*. This tissue is similar to, and continuous with, atrial muscle fiber. Therefore, any action potential that originates in the S-A node spreads into the atrium.

Cardiac fibers have the ability to automatically self-stimulate. This is particularly true with the specialized conducting network, which includes the S-A node. The S-A node is the normal pacemaker of the heart. Generating an impulse between 70 and 80 beats/min, contraction of the atrium and ventricles normally originates in the S-A node.

The uniqueness of the S-A node is related to its ability to fire off in a rhythmic fashion. This results, at least partly, from the fact that the fibers in this area are permeable to sodium ions. The S-A node has a membrane resting potential (MRP) of -60 mV, whereas ventricular fibers have an MRP of -90 mV. There is not enough of a negative voltage in the S-A node fibers to keep the calcium-sodium channels closed. This results in a constant leak until the threshold potential is reached and the cell fires off. This leakiness does not keep the fibers in a constant state of depolarization because depolarization results in a large increase in the number of potassium ions exiting the cell. This

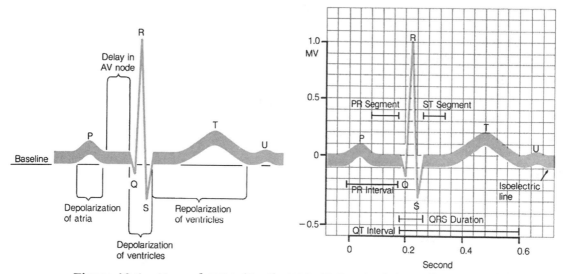

Figure 10-6.   Normal ECG. (Porth, C.M., Pathophysiology: Concepts of Altered Health States, 4th ed. Philadelphia: J.B. Lippincott, 1994, with permission.)

large number of positive ions on the outside of the cell results in an increased negativity inside the cell. This state is referred to as a state of hyperpolarization. It is responsible for driving the resting membrane potential back down to -60 mV.

Once the MRP is restored, potassium channels begin to close and the sodium again begins to leak back into the cell. Once the threshold potential is reached again, the S-A node discharges, or fires, once more.

Internodal Pathways
The S-A node fibers are continuous with the surrounding atrial muscle fibers. The electrical discharge from the S-A node spreads out into the atrial fibers and down to the A-V node. This impulse is speeded up by a number of internodal pathways (Figure 10-6). There are three bands: the interior, middle, and posterior. At this point, the action potential has spread out through the entire atrial muscle. This results in the production of a P wave in the ECG.

The Atrioventricular Node: Origin of the QRS
Located in the septal wall of the right atrium, the A-V node can discharge as the result of stimulation from an outside source. It also has its own inherent discharge rate of 40–60 beats/min. Because the inherent rate of the S-A node is greater than that of the A-V node, it overrides this discharge.

In order to allow time for emptying of the atria into the ventricles, there is a delay of the impulse traveling into the ventricles. It is the A-V node and connecting conductive fibers that delay this transmission. *Junctional fibers*, which connect normal atrial muscle fibers to the fibers of the node, are also major contributors to the delay of impulse into the A-V node. Once the electrical impulse enters the A-V node, it moves through transitional fibers and then into the bundle of His. This A-V bundle of His quickly divides into the right and left bundle branches. These branches run down their respective septal walls and then branch out into the Purkinje fibers. At this point, the impulse is transmitted by the ventricular muscle mass itself and ventricular contraction occurs.

The resulting contraction produces the QRS wave in the ECG. The atrium repolarizes at the same time the QRS is being recorded and, therefore, it is hidden (known as the atrial T wave). Once the ventricles have depolarized and contraction occurs, repolarization ensues and a T wave appears on the ECG tracing (Figure 10-6).

This entire process occurs in less than a second. The time interval between the P wave and the Q or R wave is approximately 0.16 second (PR interval). The time interval between the Q and the T wave is normally 0.35 second (Q-T interval). The QRS complex is approximately 0.08 second, as is the ST segment. Occasionally, a U wave follows the T wave; its origin is unknown. The ECG is effective at identifying abnormal cardiac rhythms and myocardial ischemia but cannot monitor pump effectiveness.

▼ MYOCARDIAL PERFORMANCE

Four major factors are responsible for determining myocardial function (Figure 10-7):

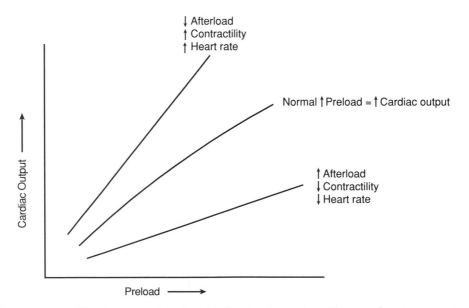

Figure 10-7.   **The impact of preload, afterload, contractility, and HR on cardiac output.**

1. Preload
2. Afterload
3. Contractility
4. Heart rate

Ventricular Function

The work required by the left and right ventricles to increase the blood pressure during each contraction is referred to as **stroke work**. The work required by the right ventricle is normally about 15% of the work required by the left ventricle. The myocardium, like any other tissue in the body, requires nutrition and oxygen. The two most important factors affecting the expenditure of energy gained from these sources are tension and time. Tension refers to the actual tension of the myocardium at the time of contraction; time refers to the length of time the tension is maintained. When the myocardium contracts, chemical energy is converted to heat and work. Approximately 20% of the efficiency of normal myocardial tissue contributes to work, whereas 80% contributes to heat loss.

The heart can only put out as much blood as it gets back. Therefore, venous return has a direct impact on cardiac output. Depending on the need, cardiac output can vary from 2 to 25 L/min. The ability of the heart to respond appropriately to changing venous return is described by Starling's law of heart. This law states that the heart will expel all of the blood that returns to it, without congestion or build up of blood in the veins.

Preload describes the degree of stretch of the myocardium at the moment before it contracts. It is the volume of blood contained in the ventricle at the end of diastole, and is also referred to as end-diastolic volume. On the right side of the heart it is the blood returning from the inferior and superior venae cavae. On the left side of the heart it is the blood returning from the four pulmonary veins. When the myocardium is stretched by an increase in venous return, it contracts with greater force. This action automatically expels the extra blood into the arteries.

The heart can also increase its contractile frequency to deal with increased venous return. Feedback from the wall of the right atrium can increase HR by as much as 30% in response to stretch.

Surprisingly, arterial pressure has little effect on cardiac output. The pressure encountered by the contracting ventricle is referred to as afterload, which is defined as the load against the myocardium during contraction. It should be kept in mind that the single most important factor determining cardiac output is the amount of blood returning to the heart (preload). (Note: This does not take into account abnormally high blood pressure, which can decrease cardiac output.)

▼ IMPACT OF MECHANICAL VENTILATION

Mechanical ventilation can reduce cardiac output by impeding venous return. Using a ventilator to move gas into the lungs can increase intrathoracic pressure and reduce venous return. If normal compensation does not occur, cardiac output will decrease. Close monitoring of cardiac function is important during mechanical ventilation, especially if the patient is already experiencing cardio-vascular instability.

▼ CARDIAC CONTROL

The heart has both sympathetic and parasympathetic (vagal) innervation. Nervous control can affect the myocardium by increasing HR (chromotropic effect) and contractility (inotropic effect). Sympathetic stimulation increases HR, whereas parasympathetic stimulation produces the opposite effect by decreasing HR (vagal stimulation).

Vagal stimulation may reduce HR by 30 beats/min and sympathetic stimulation may increase HR to over 200 beats/min. Peak cardiac output occurs at a rate of 150–250 beats/min. Within the functional limits of HR, as HR increases, the force of contraction also increases. Remember that when HR increases, there is progressively less time for ventricular refilling between contractions. The myocardium is also limited by metabolic supplies.

▼ ELECTROLYTES AND MYOCARDIAL FUNCTION

The role of sodium, potassium, and calcium in myocardial function has already been discussed. The myocardial impact of elevations and reductions in extracellular concentration of these electrolytes is an important consideration in treating a patient presenting with a cardiopulmonary complaint. We present an overview of electrolyte imbalances here and refer the reader to Chapter 12 for a more in-depth discussion.

Hypernatremia

Increased levels of extracellular sodium ions depress cardiac function. Sodium ions compete with calcium ions, reducing their effectiveness in the contractile process. Normal regulatory mechanisms make this a rare occurrence.

Hyponatremia

Decreased levels of extracellular sodium ions may even result in fibrillation (rapid, irregular contraction of atrial or ventricular muscle fibers).

Hyperkalemia

Increased levels of extracellular potassium ions result in a dilated and depressed myocardium. Abnormally high levels can actually result in an A-V block of electrical impulse. Electrical impulses do not get transmitted from the S-A node down into the ventricles. The accompanying myocardial weakness may even result in cardiac arrest. This is all because an elevated potassium level decreases MRP in the myocardium and hence contractile strength.

Hypokalemia

This condition results in excitatory changes in myocardial function. This also results in skeletal muscle weakness, a consideration in respiratory function assessment. Low levels of potassium can weaken the muscles used in breathing.

Hypercalcemia

Calcium has a tremendous impact on myocardial contractile strength. Elevated extracellular levels can result in spasmodic contractions of the myocardium.

Hypocalcemia

Reduced levels of calcium have an effect similar to hyperkalemia, causing a weak, flaccid myocardium.

▼ CORONARY BLOOD FLOW

The left coronary artery supplies the anterior and lateral part of the left ventricle, and the right coronary artery feeds most of the right ventricle and the back of the left ventricle. Coronary blood flow takes approximately 5% of the total cardiac output. In exercise, the coronary blood flow can increase three to four times to satisfy the increased need for oxygen and nutrients. Blood flow to the myocardium deteriorates during systole because of myocardial contraction and compression of the vasculature, which functions in a manner contrary to that of other tissues in the body. Figure 10-8 illlustrates the coronary arteries and veins through which this blood flow occurs.

During diastole, blood flow increases dramatically in response to muscle contraction, even if the myocardium is denervated. Oxygen consumption is also a coronary vasodilator, although the exact mechanism by which it works is not known.

Myocardial oxygen consumption increases in heart disease when the heart dilates, as in congestive heart failure, because as the heart dilates, the work required to pump a given volume of blood increases. Drugs such as epinephrine and digitalis also increase myocardial oxygen consumption, as do calcium ions. If the load on the heart exceeds blood supply, chest pain develops. This is known as angina pectoris.

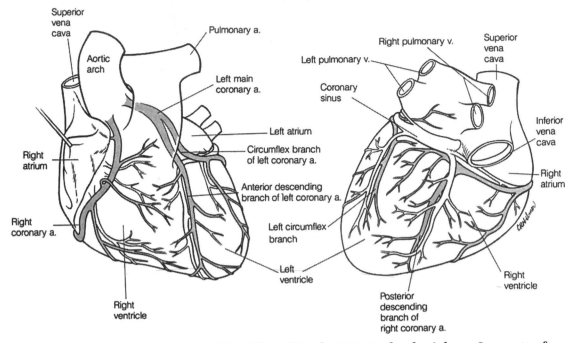

Figure 10-8.   Coronary blood flow. (Porth, C.M., Pathophysiology: Concepts of Altered Health States, 4th ed. Philadelphia: J.B. Lippincott, 1994, with permission.)

Aortic pressure is the most important determinant of coronary blood flow. Because the coronary arteries arise distally to the aortic valve, aortic pressure is extremely important to coronary blood supply. As aortic pressure increases and decreases, so does coronary blood flow. Because 75% of the oxygen contained in arterial blood is removed by the time it passes through the myocardium, blood flow is the only way of responding to increased oxygen consumption. Venous blood leaving coronary circulation contains 5 mL of oxygen per 100 mL of blood. It is easy to see the importance of aortic pressure in responding to increased myocardial demands.

Cardiac Dysrhythmias

Cardiac dysrhythmias result from abnormalities in electrophysiology. Only the specialized muscle cells such as the S-A node, internodal tracts, A-V node, bundle of His, bundle branches, and Purkinje fibers have automaticity, or the capability to generate an impulse independently. (Normal atrial or ventricular cells cannot generate an impulse independently.) Anything that can reduce the automaticity of the higher pacemaker sites can result in the movement of the pacemaker to a lower center. This process is considered passive and can result from any factor with vagal influences.

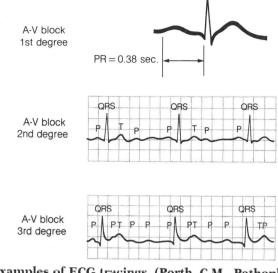

Figure 10-9.   Examples of ECG tracings. (Porth, C.M., Pathophysiology: Concepts of Altered Health States, 4th ed. Philadelphia: J.B. Lippincott, 1994, with permission.)

Ectopic foci are centers of automaticity outside the S-A node. Sympathetic influences, myocardial ischemia (inadequate flow of blood to the heart), **hypercapnia** (increased carbon dioxide in blood), and **hypoxia** (decreased oxygen concentration in inspired air) all can cause ectopic foci. Reentry is a term often used to describe impaired conduction. This is a problem often resulting from myocardial injury, such as myocardial ischemia or infarction. The result is a delayed or slowed conduction reentering, which causes an abnormal heart rhythm. The set of ECG tracings in Figure 10-9 shows how various cardiac conditions can alter the QRS complex.

▼ CONCLUSION

The heart provides the driving force necessary to push blood out into the body and back. In terms of respiration, oxygen delivery and carbon dioxide removal are limited by cardiovascular function. Knowing the limitations of gas transport requires a comprehensive understanding of the heart and its physiological influences. This chapter has described the fundamental concepts of heart function from myocardial physiology to control and outside influences. It is important to understand that this is only the foundation needed to develop a more comprehensive view of cardiopulmonary care. From this foundation it is possi-

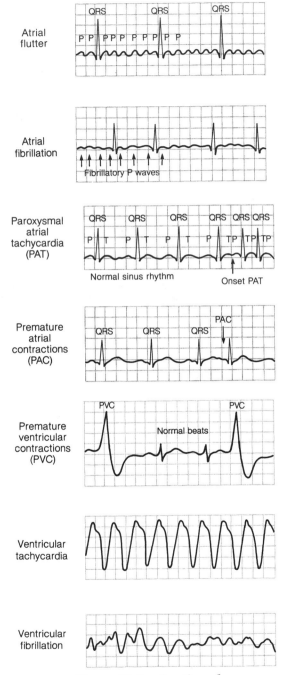

Atrial flutter

Atrial fibrillation

Paroxysmal atrial tachycardia (PAT)

Premature atrial contractions (PAC)

Premature ventricular contractions (PVC)

Ventricular tachycardia

Ventricular fibrillation

Figure 10-9.   Continued

ble to move on to explore the "beneficiary" of the heart's rhythmic pumping: systemic circulation.

❖ Review Questions

1. The heart contains
   i. atrial muscle.
   ii. skeletal muscle.
   iii. ventricular muscle.
   iv. striated muscle fibers 3 μm long.
   v. excitatory fibers.

   a. i, ii
   b. ii, iii
   c. i, iii, v
   d. iii, iv, v
   e. ii, iv, v

2. Ventricular muscle cells in the heart
   i. are very complex fibers compared with atrial muscles.
   ii. have a shorter refractory period than atrial muscle.
   iii. contract only weakly.
   iv. may function as an ideal conduction network.
   v. can contract at a higher rate than atrial muscle.

   a. i, ii
   b. ii, iii
   c. iii, iv
   d. ii, iv, v
   e. i, ii, iv, v

3. Transverse tubules in heart muscle
   i. are a channel-like system connecting the sarcolemma.
   ii. run along and across myocardial cells.
   iii. contain the cell actin and myosin.
   iv. extend into the myocardial fiber.
   v. are filled with interstitial fluid.

   a. i, ii
   b. ii, iii
   c. iii, iv, v
   d. i, ii, iii, v
   e. ii, iii, iv, v

4. Normal cardiac muscle has a resting membrane potential of approximately (in millivolts)
   a. +20.
   b. +10.
   c. −40.
   d. −60.
   e. −90.

5. Phase 2 of the myocardial action potential represents
   a. delay in repolarization.
   b. rapid depolarization.
   c. absolute refractory period.
   d. rapid repolarization.
   e. spontaneous diastolic depolarization.
6. The cardiac cycle is
   i. the time from the beginning of one contraction to the beginning of the next.
   ii. both systole and diastole.
   iii. resulting in blood pressure changes.
   iv. responsible for variations in atrial and ventricular heart rate.
   v. responsible for heart rate changes seen during rest and exercise.

   a. i, ii
   b. ii, iii
   c. i, ii, iii
   d. ii, iv, v
   e. i, ii, iv, v
7. In systemic terms, the dicrotic notch seen within a pressure waveform of the heart results from
   a. closure of the aortic valve.
   b. closure of the pulmonic valve.
   c. contraction of the aorta.
   d. contraction of the pulmonary artery.
   e. semilunar valve closure.
8. Pulsatile waves have been recorded in the major veins and are referred to as
   i. a waves.
   ii. b waves.
   iii. c waves.
   iv. v waves.
   v. z waves.

   a. i, ii, iii
   b. ii, iii, iv
   c. i, iii, iv
   d. ii, iv, v
   e. ii, iii, iv, v
9. The third heart sound is believed to result from
   a. aortic opening.
   b. closure of the aorta.
   c. contraction of the atrium.
   d. rapid filling of the ventricles.
   e. contraction of the ventricles.

10. The PR interval is approximately (in seconds)
    a. 0.08.
    b. 0.16.
    c. 0.35.
    d. 0.42.
    e. 0.50.

11

CIRCULATION

Matthews LR: CARDIOPULMONARY ANATOMY AND PHYSIOLOGY. © 1996 Lippincott–Raven Publishers.

OBJECTIVES

1. Review the anatomy of the circulatory system and explain its function.
2. Identify the vessels within the circulatory system in terms of diameter and linings.
3. Describe the normal arterial and venous pressures from the aorta to the vena cava.
4. Define normal venous blood pressure and mean arterial pressure.
5. Explain how blood is distributed throughout the various body systems and discuss how blood flow is regulated.
6. Describe hemodynamics in terms of pressure flow and resistance.
7. Describe the autonomic control of circulation.
8. Define Pouseuille's law in terms of blood flow in a vessel.
9. Define conductance and describe its function.
10. Define critical closing pressure and vessel diameter.
11. Explain sympathetic nervous control of the arterial and venous vasculature.
12. Describe central nervous control of the arterial and venous vasculature.
13. Name the vascular reflexes and explain their functions.
14. List the general causes of shock and describe each.
15. Explain the metabolic function of circulation.
16. Define anabolism and catabolism.
17. Discuss the basic concept of recommended daily allowance.

The cardiovascular system consists of the heart (which we addressed in the previous chapter), blood vessels (arteries, arterioles, capillaries, veins, and venules), and the lymphatic system. The circulation that is routed through this system is a continuous circuit, which is to say that blood put out by the right side of the heart into the lungs (pulmonary circulation) must ultimately be put out by the left side of the heart into systemic circulation. Figure 11-1 depicts the blood vessels categorized into arteries and veins; Figure 11-2 shows a simplification of the pulmonary and systemic circulations.

Each region of the body can control its own blood flow to meet its particular needs, which include

1. obtaining oxygen and nutrients.
2. liberating carbon dioxide,
3. expelling hydrogen ions.
4. maintaining a balance of electrolytes.
5. receiving or expelling hormones.

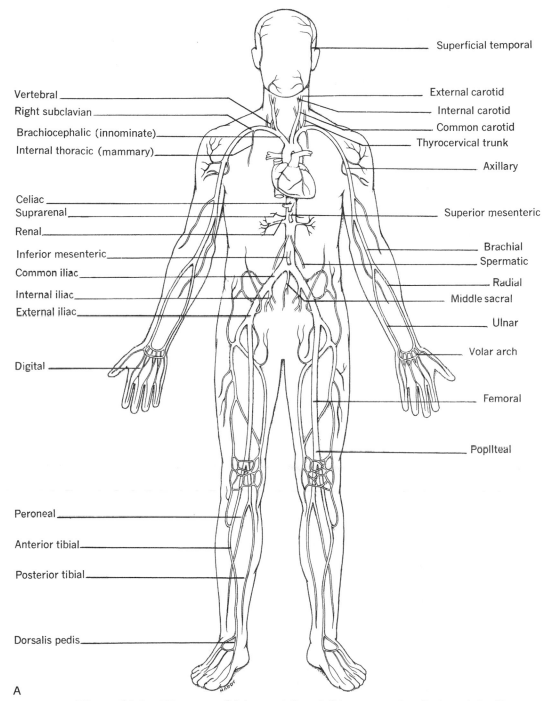

Superficial temporal

Vertebral

Right subclavian

Brachiocephalic (innominate)

Internal thoracic (mammary)

External carotid

Internal carotid

Common carotid

Thyrocervical trunk

Axillary

Celiac

Suprarenal

Renal

Superior mesenteric

Inferior mesenteric

Common iliac

Brachial

Spermatic

Radial

Internal iliac

External iliac

Middle sacral

Ulnar

Volar arch

Digital

Femoral

Popliteal

Peroneal

Anterior tibial

Posterior tibial

Dorsalis pedis

A

Figure 11-1.   Diagram of (a) arterial and (b) venous circulation. (Chaffee, E.E. and Lytle, I.M., Basic Physiology and Anatomy, 4th ed. Philadelphia: J.B. Lippincott, 1980, with permission.)

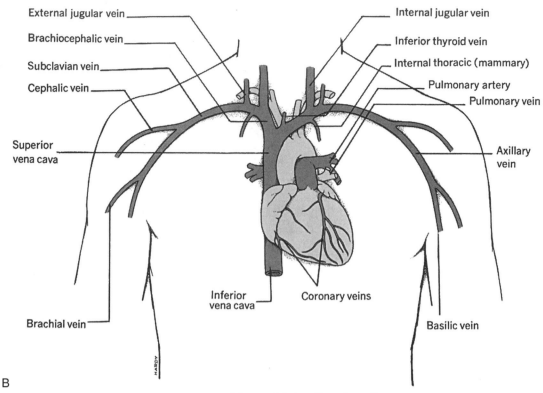

External jugular vein

Brachiocephalic vein

Subclavian vein

Cephalic vein

Internal jugular vein

Inferior thyroid vein

Internal thoracic (mammary)

Pulmonary artery

Pulmonary vein

Superior vena cava

Axillary vein

Inferior vena cava

Coronary veins

Brachial vein

Basilic vein

B

Figure 11-1.   Continued

▼ CIRCULATORY ANATOMY

Arteries and Veins

The term "artery" is used to describe vessels leaving the heart, and the term "vein" is applied to those vessels that return to the heart.

Arteries are elastic, muscular tubes that gradually become smaller and smaller until they become arterioles, at which point they enter the microscopic capillary network. The veins are responsible for conducting blood from the capillary network back to the heart (Figure 11-3). Capable of constricting or expanding, the veins also serve as a variable reservoir that can respond to body needs. Table 11-1 lists the blood vessels and their respective diameters.

The Arteries

The arteries consist of three coats, or layers, of tissue (Figure 11-3):

1. The inner layer (tunica intima) is an endothelium, resting on an elastic membrane.
2. The middle layer (tunica media) occupies the bulk of the arterial wall. It contains elastic connective tissue and smooth muscle.
3. The outer layer (tunica externa) is made up mostly of connective tissue, giving strength to the arterial wall.

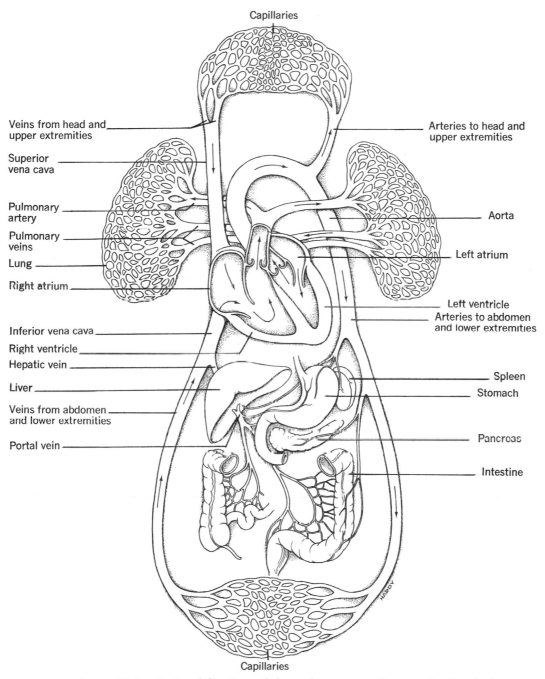

Capillaries

Veins from head and
upper extremities

Superior
vena cava

Pulmonary
artery

Pulmonary
veins

Lung

Right atrium

Inferior vena cava

Right ventricle

Hepatic vein

Liver

Veins from abdomen
and lower extremities

Portal vein

Arteries to head and
upper extremities

Aorta

Left atrium

Left ventricle
Arteries to abdomen
and lower extremities

Spleen

Stomach

Pancreas

Intestine

Capillaries

**Figure 11-2.   A simplification of the pulmonary and systemic circulation.
(Chaffee, E.E. and Lytle, I.M., Basic Physiology and Anatomy, 4th ed.
Philadelphia: J.B. Lippincott, 1980, with permission.)**

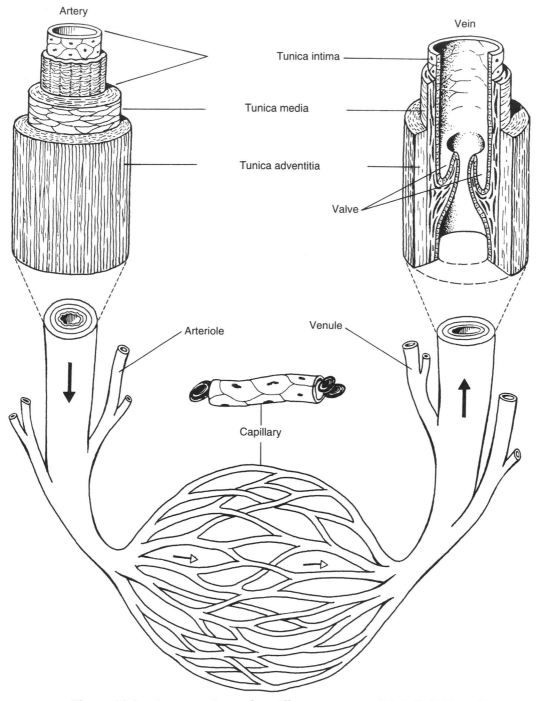

Figure 11-3.   Artery, vein, and capillary structure. (McCall, R.E. and Tankersley, C.M., Phlebotomy Essentials. Philadelphia: J.B. Lippincott, 1993, with permission.)

TABLE 11-1   Cross-Sectional Area of the Vasculature

Vessel	Diameter (cm²)
Aorta	2.5
Small artery	20
Arterioles	40
Capillaries	2,500
Venules	250
Small veins	80
Vena cava	8

The large arteries have two major functions:

1. to serve as a conduit for transport of blood to the tissues
2. to serve as a high pressure reservoir during diastole

Oxygen is transported from the lung to the tissues in about 10 seconds. The elastic nature of the arteries is important because it prevents blood pressure from abnormally increasing during ventricular contraction. It also allows blood flow to move continuously with intermittent pumping from the heart.

The Small Arteries and Arterioles

Blood flow to various organ systems in the body is controlled almost entirely by the degree of contraction or dilation of the small arteries and arterioles. The strong muscular walls of these vessels are their most important feature.

The Veins

These vessels also can constrict and enlarge. Acting as a large reservoir for blood, this system can constrict and propel blood forward by means of the venous pump. This low-pressure system contains a series of check valves responsible for ensuring that blood flows in one direction only, back toward the heart. Like the arteries, the veins have three coats or layers: the tunica intima, tunica media, and tunica externa. However, in the veins the tunica media consists of only a thin layer of smooth muscle and a few elastic fibers (Figure 11-3).

▼ ARTERIAL AND VENOUS BLOOD PRESSURES

Normal Arterial Blood Pressure

Normal arterial blood pressure varies with age, gradually increasing over the years. At birth, pressure is approximately 80 mmHg systolic and 60 mmHg diastolic. It averages 120 mmHg systolic and 80 mmHg diastolic throughout life. In later years, systolic pressure may approach 200 mmHg.

Systemic and pulmonary systolic pressure results from contraction of the ventricles, whereas diastolic pressure is a result of arterial smooth muscle relaxation.

Normal Venous Blood Pressure

The pressure at the beginning of the venous system is approximately 10 mmHg and it drops to 0 mmHg by the time it reaches the right side of the heart. The pressure in the right atrium is commonly referred to as **central venous pressure**. This pressure is influenced by three factors: the effectiveness of the right atrium at pumping blood into the right ventricle, the amount of blood returning to the heart via the inferior and superior venae cavae, and right ventricular function.

Mean Arterial Pressure

The mean, or average, blood pressure in humans is approximately 95 mmHg. This value is important because it is the mean arterial pressure that provides the driving force for tissue blood flow (peripheral perfusion).

▼ CIRCULATING BLOOD VOLUME

Approximately 65% of the total blood volume (5 L in total, which breaks down to 3 L of plasma and 2 L of red blood cells) is contained on the venous side of the circulation; 15% of it occupies the arteries; and 10% can be found in pulmonary circulation (Figure 11-4). The remainder is contained in the heart and capillary

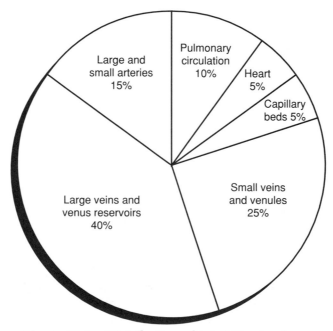

Figure 11-4.   Distribution of total blood volume.

beds (see Chapter 10). The functional part of this system is in the capillary bed, yet only about 5% of the total blood volume is contained in this area at any given point in time. The capillary beds are only 0.3–1.0 mm in length and width. Given that blood flows through them at 0.3 mm/sec, it takes 1–3 seconds for diffusion to occur.

A decrease in blood volume can result in a decrease in blood pressure. Normally, compensatory mechanisms (i.e., pressure sensors in the *carotid sinuses*, a dilated area in the bifurcation in the carotid artery) prompt a constriction of the venous reservoir. Constricting the venous reservoir compensates for the blood loss and maintains blood pressure. As much as a 20% volume loss can occur before a decrease in pressure results. Blood reservoirs exist in the spleen, liver, large abdominal veins, and skin. Indeed, one of the first indicators that compensation is occurring is a reduction of blood flow to the skin.

The heart and lungs also can act as reservoirs. When stimulated, the heart can reduce in size and contribute up to 100 mL of blood. If pulmonary pressures decrease, the pulmonary vasculature can constrict and contribute another 200 mL to the needed blood volume.

High blood volume can result in an elevation of blood pressure and congestive heart failure.

▼ HEMODYNAMICS

Pressure, Flow, and Resistance

Blood flow throughout the pulmonary and systemic circulation depends on the pressure difference across the system and the vascular resistance to flow:

$$\dot{Q} = P/R$$

where $\dot{Q}$ = blood flow, P = pressure, and R = resistance.

Consequently, if a given cardiac output is required with a given vascular resistance, the heart must generate the necessary pressure (it also follows that the heart must work harder as vascular resistance is increased):

$$P = \dot{Q} \times R$$

$\dot{Q}$ is generated by the heart and is dependent on venous return. Blood flow is generally expressed in liters per minute (see Chapter 10).

Resistance is described in terms of the amount of pressure required to move a given volume of blood (flow or cardiac output) through a vessel:

$$R = P/\dot{Q}$$

Blood Pressure

Generally, we use mmHg when describing blood pressure. Figure 11-5 shows the pulsatile force generated by the heart as it contracts and relaxes. The difference between systolic and diastolic pressure is known as **pulse pressure**. This

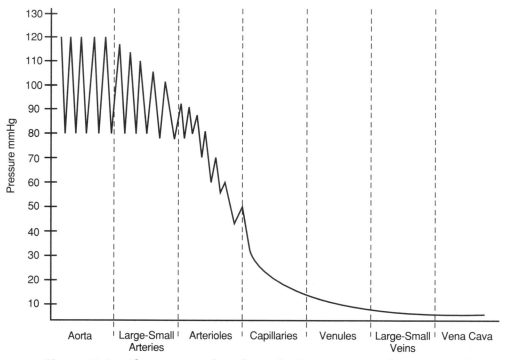

Figure 11-5. The pressure drop from the largest artery, the aorta, to the largest vein, the vena cava.

pulse pressure is significant in that it is a representation of ventricular stroke volume and the compliance of the arteries into which it pumps. As stroke volume increases, the pressure increases. However, if the arteries are compliant (distensible), this pressure increase will be minimized. The reverse is also true: if the arteries are stiff (i.e., low compliance arteriosclerosis), the pressure increase will be great.

Pressure Wave

The pressure pulsation generated by the heart is not immediately transmitted to the periphery. The pressure is generated outward in a wave that moves faster and faster as it travels from the aorta into the major arteries and then even farther into the smaller arteries. This pressure pulse is up to 100 times the speed of the actual blood flow, meaning that the pressure pulse is felt long before the blood reaches the point of palpation.

As a wave of pressure moves outward, it encounters less compliant, or stiffer, vessels. Just as a water wave returns after striking an object, the pressure wave in the arterial tree moves back toward the heart. This backward pressure wave accumulates with the forward pressure wave, increasing the pulse pressure. This phenomenon can result in a significant increase in pulse pressure when monitoring pressure in a peripheral artery. Systolic pressure can be increased by greater than 20% and diastolic pressure can be reduced by as much as 10%.

Pulsus paradoxus describes a clinical manifestation resulting in a strong then weak radial pulse. This variation is synchronized with the breathing pattern. Cardiac output and pulse strength are affected by intrathoracic pressures generated during inspiration and expiration. If intrathoracic pressures are abnormal, inspiration temporarily reduces venous return to the heart and decreases stroke volume, and thus pulse strength. This may occur in cases of status asthmaticus. Myocardial compression (cardiac tamponade) can also affect pulsatile strength.

Pulsus alternans is characterized by a weak heart beat that is followed by a strong heart beat. This may be a result of abnormal rhythms or oscillations in circulating blood volume caused by enlarged ventricles.

Regulation of Blood Flow

There are different blood supplies required for the various organ systems, depending on their metabolic requirements. Table 11-2 shows, in decreasing need, the various organs' blood flow requirements at rest.

The body can vary blood supply to the organs according to need. Either an increase in the need for oxygen and nutrients or a decrease in the availability of the same can result in an increased blood supply.

Two theories exist to describe this phenomenon: the theory of vasodilation and the theory of oxygen demand.

The theory of vasodilation suggests that as tissue metabolic rate begins to increase, chemical mediators are released that are responsible for vasodilation. This results in an increase in blood flow. Although adenosine seems to be the most likely single mediator responsible, a combination of factors is more likely to achieve this effect.

The theory of oxygen demand suggests that a deficiency of oxygen and other nutrients causes vascular dilation and hence an increase in blood supply.

Whether it is the vasodilation theory, oxygen demand theory, or a combination of the two that is responsible for vasodilation, the fact still remains that blood is regulated according to metabolic demand.

TABLE 11-2 Distribution of Blood Flow	
Organ	% of Total Cardiac Output
Liver	25%
Kidneys	20%
Brain	15%
Muscle	15%
Skin	5%
Bone	5%
Other organ systems	15%

▼ AUTONOMIC CONTROL OF CIRCULATION

Sympathetic innervation is significant in its impact on the regulation of blood flow. It most commonly functions by increasing smooth muscle tone and, hence, increasing the resistance to blood flow. Sympathetic innervation can also result in smooth muscle dilation.

Vasoconstriction and Dilation

Resistance to Blood Flow

The resistance to blood flow is commonly expressed in dyne seconds per centimeter[5]. When using these units, resistance can be calculated with the following formula:

$$\text{Resistance} = [1{,}330 \times \text{(i)mmHg}]/\text{(ii)mL/sec}$$

where (i) = the pressure difference across the circulatory system from arterial to venous (normally, this value is approximately 100 mmHg systemic and 15 mmHg pulmonary); (ii) = the blood flow through the system (the normal value is approximately 5 L/min, or 83 mL/sec); and 1,330 = the factor used to convert mmHg to dyne per centimeter[2].

Plugging in the standard values, we can compute systemic vascular resistance to be

$$[1{,}330 \times 100]/83 = 1{,}600 \text{ dynes sec/cm}^{-5}$$

Pulmonary vascular resistance is equal to

$$[1{,}330 \times 15]/83 = 240 \text{ dyne sec/cm}^{-5}$$

Notice the dramatic difference in resistance when comparing systemic and pulmonary vascular resistance. Resistance in the pulmonary vasculature is approximately six to seven times lower than systemic vascular resistance.

These values are often standardized to include body surface area (BSA). This takes into account the differences in body size from one individual to another. In this case, the value is referred to as the **vascular resistance index** and is expressed as dynes seconds/cm^{-5}/M^{-2} (the final value is the measurement of body BSA). Vascular resistance has an indirect effect on blood flow. With a given pressure difference across the circulatory system as resistance increases, blood flow decreases.

Poiseuille's law states that the resistance to blood flow in a vessel is directly proportional to the blood viscosity and length of the vessel, but it is inversely proportional to the fourth power of the radius. This illustrates the importance of vascular tone. With a given pressure difference across the vessels, blood flow is increased 16-fold if the diameter is cut in half.

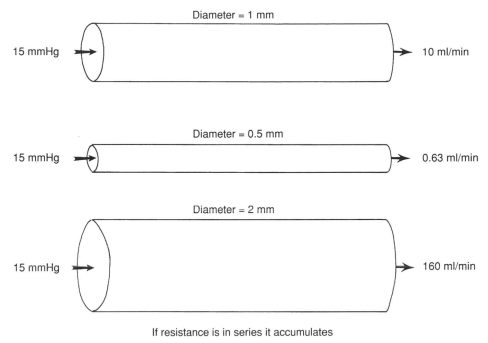

Figure 11-6. A schematic representation of the effects of vasculature tone on blood flow. (Top) Normal. (Middle) Increased tone. (Bottom) Decreased tone.

Effects of Vasculature Tone on Blood Flow

Figure 11-6 illustrates the effects of vasculature tone on blood flow. If resistance is in series, it accumulates:

$$R_{series} = R_1 + R_2 + R_3$$

If resistance is parallel, it decreases as more vessels are added. This is because the cross-sectional area is increased when more blood vessels are added.

Conductance

Conductance is another term commonly used to describe blood flow through a vessel. It is described as the reciprocal of resistance. In other words, as resistance increases, conductance decreases. Conductance is directly related to blood flow.

$$Conductance = 1/resistance$$

Critical Closing Pressure and Vessel Diameter

An increase or decrease in pressure has a direct effect on the diameter of the vessel. As blood pressure increases, so does the diameter of the vessel; the reverse is also true. As blood pressure changes, both the force pushing the blood and the diameter of the vessel change.

If blood pressure is increased, then the force pushing on the blood is increased and the diameter increases as an expression of reduced resistance. This results in an exponential increase in blood flow as pressure is increased.

The muscular tone of an artery can collapse a vessel if the pressure is not sufficient to keep it open. This pressure is known as the **critical closing pressure**. When pressure is too low and the vessels become very small, blood cells can actually become lodged in the pathway and obstruct further movement of blood flow.

Sympathetic Nervous Control

Sympathetic nerve fibers are distributed throughout the arterial and venous vasculature. Stimulation of these fibers results in vasoconstriction, increased resistance, and changes in blood flow. When veins are stimulated to constrict, volume reserve is reduced and there is an increase in blood flow back to the heart, which has the effect of increasing cardiac output. Sympathetic stimulation to the heart also results in an increased heart rate, further increasing cardiac output.

Continuous stimulation from sympathetic nervous fibers is necessary to maintain smooth muscle tone and hence regulate blood pressure. Most blood vessels in the body are constricted to 50% of their completely dilated size to allow for modulation of blood flow. In other words, the vessels stand ready to accommodate both an increase and a decrease in resistance as needed. The neurotransmitter responsible for vasoconstriction is norepinephrine. It is secreted at all sympathetic neuroeffector sites and, when secreted into the circulation, it usually causes vasoconstriction. In fact, the adrenal medullae continuously secrete epinephrine and norepinephrine, contributing significantly to overall smooth muscle tone and basal regulation of blood pressure. Removal of this stimulation results in reduced blood pressure.

Parasympathetic innervation has almost no effect on vasculature. Its impact on circulation is almost entirely through its effect on the heart. The vagus nerve is a parasympathetic fiber that, among other things, runs from the medulla to the heart (cranial nerve 10). This nerve causes a significant decrease in heart rate and a minor decrease in myocardial contractility.

Central Nervous System Control of Blood Pressure

The vasomotor center is located in the lower pons and the medulla. Sympathetic fibers originate in this area of the brain. This center can either increase or inhibit sympathetic output. In this way, vascular resistance can be controlled or regulated. This center also can control heart activity. Contractility and heart rate can be increased or decreased through this center. Sympathetic nerve stimulation results in cardiac stimulation, and vagus nerve stimulation results in inhibition.

The *hypothalamus* (brain region that integrates sympathetic and parasympathetic activities) and the *cerebral cortex* also can control the heart and vasculature through the vasomotor center. In fact, it is the hypothalamus that is responsible for flight or fright response: stimulation of this area results in vasodilation and increased blood flow to the muscles, vasoconstriction to other regions of the body (i.e., bowels), increased heart rate and contractility, glycogenesis, and general conscious excitement.

Remember that the primary determinant of cardiac output is venous return (preload).

▼ REFLEXES

Baroreceptors

These receptors are located in the walls of the major arteries. When blood pressure increases, baroreceptors are stimulated to direct their influence into the vasomotor center, causing inhibition of sympathetic output. This reflex is necessary for blood pressure stabilization.

Blood Volume Reflexes

These receptors are located in the major veins and the right and left atria. Stretching them increases urinary output by stimulating the kidneys through the vasomotor center and reducing secretion of antidiuretic hormone through effects on the hypothalamus.

Temperature Reflexes

If body temperature increases (hyperthermia), the hypothalamus is stimulated to dilate blood vessels in the skin. This dilation aids in releasing heat from the body and reducing core temperature. The reverse also occurs in the face of hypothermia. Blood is shunted to the body core in an attempt to conserve heat.

Humoral Influences

Circulating chemicals or substances can have a significant impact on circulation throughout the body. Among the substances that can cause vasoconstriction are

1. epinephrine and norepinephrine.
2. angiotensin.
3. vasopressin.

Among the substances that can cause vasodilation are

1. bradykinin.
2. histamine.

3. serotonin.
4. prostaglandins.

Increased calcium and decreased potassium, magnesium, sodium, plasma glucose concentrations, and hydrogen ion concentration all result in vasoconstriction.

In the lung, **hypercarbia** (increased amount of carbon dioxide in the blood) and elevated hydrogen ion concentration result in vasoconstriction. **Hypoxia** also results in pulmonary vasoconstriction. This results in selective distribution of blood to the better ventilated and oxygenated regions of the lung. In most tissues, elevated carbon dioxide results in only a moderate vasodilation, except for the brain, where carbon dioxide can significantly dilate vasculature. This response is necessary to remove any excess carbon dioxide in the brain. **Hypocapnia** and **alkalosis** cause cerebral vascular constriction and reduced intracranial pressure (ICP). It should be kept in mind that this constriction can cause cerebral hypoxia and a reduction in the supply of glucose. If hyperventilation is used to reduce ICP, the arterial-venous oxygen content difference across the head should be monitored closely.

In the lung, blood must be distributed to regions that are well ventilated and oxygenated and turned away from areas of consolidation.

When lung disease results in a considerable amount of disruption in blood flow through the lung, pulmonary vascular resistance is commonly increased. If the work imposed on the right side of the heart is prolonged, right ventricular hypertrophy and failure (cor pulmonale) may occur.

Chronic bronchitis (chronic obstructive pulmonary disease) commonly results in a cascade of events, which ultimately lead to pulmonary hypertension and right ventricular failure (Figure 11-7).

Chronic lung disease results in long-term hypoxemia, which results in

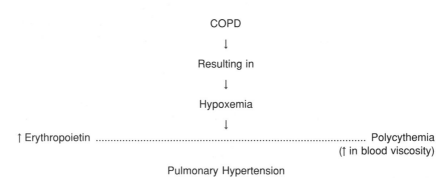

Figure 11-7.   Schematic representation of the cascade of events that lead from chronic bronchitis to right ventricular failure.

pulmonary vascular constriction and increased pulmonary vascular resistance. This hypoxemia also stimulates an increase in the production of red blood cells (RBCs), causing polycythemia. More RBCs in the blood increase the blood's viscosity and therefore further increases the load placed on the heart. The ultimate result of right ventricular heart failure is the worst-case result.

▼ SHOCK

Shock describes a general circulatory deficiency resulting in inadequate delivery of nutrients and oxygen to the cells. The general causes include the following abnormalities:

1. Decreased cardiac output
2. Septicemia
3. Hypovolemia
4. Neurogenic shock
5. Anaphylaxis

Decreased Cardiac Output

This condition results in a general decrease in the delivery of oxygen and nutrients to the cells. Anything that results in a decrease in the ability of the heart to pump can result in shock, commonly referred to as **cardiogenic shock**. It may be a result of myocardial infarction, valve dysfunction, dysrhythmias, and a number of other abnormalities. Reduced venous return also obviously reduces cardiac output.

Septicemia

Sometimes called "blood poisoning," septicemia refers to an infection that is no longer localized in one region of the body. The infection has now overcome the body's defense mechanisms and has become a widespread systemic infection, spreading through the bloodstream. In about one half of cases, the associated vasodilation, high metabolic rate, and high body temperature cause an increase in cardiac output. The peripheral vasodilation and increased body temperature has often given this form of shock the name "warm shock." The infection infiltrates the circulatory system, eventually resulting in circulatory collapse. Abnormalities in oxygen use, as a result of the septicemia, may make the assessment of hypoxia difficult.

Hypovolemia

Hemorrhagic shock is the most common cause of this general reduction in blood volume and venous return. As long as the normal compensatory mechanisms are intact, up to 30% of the patient's blood volume can be lost without death.

Neurogenic Shock

This condition is the result of a significant increase in vascular capacity through the loss of vasomotor tone. When the veins dilate, blood pools and venous return to the heart is reduced, which in turn reduces cardiac output. This reduced cardiac output further aggravates the problem.

Anaphylaxis

This allergic reaction results in reduced cardiac output and blood pressure. Bronchospasm and reduced pulmonary ventilation also result.

▼ METABOLIC FUNCTIONS OF CIRCULATION

The circulatory system is responsible for supplying nutrients and removing wastes from cells throughout the body. Adenosine triphosphate (ATP) is the raw substance that can be used by the cells of the body for various functions. ATP is the energy source that forms peptide linkages between amino acids to build proteins. These are the building blocks of the body. ATP is used in the synthesis of almost all substances in the body and is required for muscular contraction.

Because of the importance of ATP, the body must be able to store this substance in the form of phosphocreatine, although the production of phosphocreatine and then its return to ATP requires an energy expenditure itself.

The production of ATP requires the metabolism of carbohydrates, lipids, and proteins. Each substance is metabolized in distinct ways, as outlined in the following subsections.

Carbohydrate Metabolism

The end result of digesting carbohydrates is primarily the production of glucose (approximately 80%). The remaining product is converted to glucose entirely by the liver. Remember that insulin is necessary for glucose transport across most cell walls, with the exception of liver and brain cells. Once inside the cell, glucose can be used immediately for energy or it can be stored in the form of glycogen. The formation of glycogen requires the interaction of several enzymes. Lactic acid, glycerol, and pyruvic acid all can be converted into glucose and then to glycogen in a process known as **glycogenesis**.

To use the glycogen, phosphorylase must be activated by epinephrine (released by the adrenal medulla) or glucagon (released by the pancreas). These hormones increase the formation of cyclic adenosine monophosphate. This intracellular substance then activates phosphorylase, resulting in the production of glucose. The respiratory quotient for carbohydrate metabolism in the presence of oxygen is 1.0, meaning that carbon dioxide production is equal to oxygen consumption:

$$\text{Respiratory quotient} = CO_2 \text{ production}/O_2 \text{ consumption}$$

$$= 250 \text{ mL/min}/250 \text{ mL/min}$$

$$= 1.0$$

If oxygen is not available for the metabolic process using glucose, an anaerobic pathway is taken and glucose is converted to pyruvic acid. When pyruvic acid is in excess, it is stored as lactic acid. This process produces about 20 times less energy than when oxygen is available and its end product, lactic acid, cannot be removed from the body through the lungs. Remember, carbon dioxide is the normal end product of aerobic metabolism and can be exhaled via the lungs. The lactic acid can build up and lead to metabolic acidosis.

Lipid Metabolism

These chemical compounds are commonly known as fat and referred to as triglycerides, phospholipids, or cholesterol. They are long-chain hydrocarbon organic acids.

Triglycerides

Except for the brain, all body tissues can use fatty acids interchangeably with glucose. Carbohydrates (glucose) are often ingested and stored as triglycerides. Carbohydrates must be converted to fat for storage. Most cells in the body have a limited ability to store carbohydrates, and fat stores many more calories per weight than do carbohydrates. When more protein is ingested than required for immediate use, it also can be converted and stored as triglycerides. However, this conversion is not without cost; energy is lost in this process (i.e., glucose loses about 15% of its potential energy production when converted to triglycerides).

Phospholipids

These compounds are required for the production or function of lipoproteins, thromboplastin, sphingomyelin, cell membranes, and a number of specific chemical reactions.

Cholesterol

The most important use of cholesterol is in the formation of cholic acid. Cholic acid is used in combination with other substances in the liver to form bile salts and assist digestion and absorption of fats.

When triglycerides are used for the production of energy, their respiratory quotient is approximately 0.7. This means that less carbon dioxide is produced for a given volume of oxygen consumed. When glucose is used, 10 mL of oxygen metabolized produces 10 mL of carbon dioxide. In the case of fat, 10 mL of oxygen used produces 7 mL of carbon dioxide. The normal respiratory quotient is 0.8, indicating that under normal circumstances the majority of available energy is derived from free fatty acids (fatty acids combined with albumin).

Protein Metabolism

The vast majority of the body's structures are made up of proteins, which are themselves made up of various combinations of amino acids. Some proteins may contain as few as 20 amino acids, whereas others have more than 500.

The three major plasma proteins are albumin, globulin, and fibrinogen. Albumin prevents plasma loss by providing colloid osmotic pressure and is responsible for carrying fatty acids throughout the body. Globulin's most important function is immunity (natural and acquired) against invading organisms. Fibrinogen is necessary in the clotting process for leak repair in the circulatory system.

Essential and nonessential amino acids are present in the body. Essential amino acids must be present in the diet because they are either not synthesized in the body or are synthesized in quantities too small for survival. The nonessential amino acids are as important functionally as essential amino acids, but it is not essential that they be in our diet. If we do not eat protein, body proteins begin to break down. Approximately 30 g of protein per day will be lost in this manner. Normally, the body uses carbohydrates and fats for energy production. This may prolong survival during severe stress or starvation. However, it is not advantageous to long-term survival because it depletes the fundamental building blocks of the body. When the body is metabolizing protein, the respiratory quotient is 0.8 (Table 11-3).

Lipids and proteins produce less carbon dioxide than do carbohydrates because they produce more hydrogen ions when they are metabolized. Therefore, more oxygen molecules combine with these hydrogen ions to produce water and less oxygen combines with carbon to produce carbon dioxide.

Respiratory exchange ratio describes the exchange of carbon dioxide and oxygen in the lung. The moment-to-moment respiratory exchange ratio and respiratory quotient can vary significantly. But over a period of time, they must eventually average out and be equal to each other. If this does not happen, either a build-up or a depletion of carbon dioxide develops.

TABLE 11-3 CO_2 Production

	RQ	CO_2 Production/min	Energy Production
Carbohydrates	1.0	250 mL	4 Kcal/g
Lipids	0.7	175 mL	9 Kcal/g
Proteins	0.8	200 mL	4 Kcal/g

RQ, respiratory quotient. Oxygen consumption: 250 mL/min.

Anabolism and Catabolism

Metabolism consists of two phases: anabolism and catabolism. **Anabolism** describes the phase of metabolism responsible for the storage and synthesis of cell constituents. This process requires energy. **Catabolism** describes the breakdown of molecules required for the necessary energy production.

Recommended Daily Allowance

Normal metabolic function requires over 40 nutrients daily. The Recommended Daily Allowance (RDA) describes the necessary nutritional intake required to meet the needs of an average healthy individual. Generally, it represents 200–600% of the minimum requirement. Normal metabolic function requires the ingestion of proteins, fats, carbohydrates, vitamins, and minerals. Many hospitalized patients are malnourished. In particular, critical care patients must be monitored closely and necessary nutritional needs should be provided. Ventilation function can be adversely affected by a lack of the necessary metabolic components for energy production and structural cell maintenance.

▼ CONCLUSION

This chapter has described the system of connecting tubes used to transport blood around the body. The structure of arteries, arterioles, venules, and veins was described to promote an understanding of how blood pressure is maintained. The importance of maintaining blood volume also was discussed. The interrelationship of all of the above-mentioned factors is known as hemodynamics; a thorough understanding of this area is necessary for in-depth understanding of cardiopulmonary function.

The monitoring and analysis of these factors was also described to provide the student with an appreciation for a normally functioning system, which provides an accurate baseline against which to measure function once disease ensues. The important neurological factors were also presented to illustrate the ins and outs of day-to-day regulatory mechanisms. Finally, the metabolic function of circulation was described to show its importance in supplying the body's nutritional needs.

❖ Review Questions

1. The cross-sectional area of the aorta is approximately (cm²)
   a. 2.5.
   b. 20.
   c. 40.
   d. 80.
   e. 100.

2. Which of the following are layers of an artery?
   i.   Tunica intima
   ii. Tunica media
   iii. Tunica extravenous
   iv. Tunica externa
   v.   Arterious muscularous

   a. i, ii, iii
   b. iii, iv, v
   c. i, ii, iv
   d. ii, iv, v
   e. i, ii, v
3. Which of the following pressures is most important in providing the driving force for tissue blood flow?
   a. Systolic arterial pressure
   b. Diastolic arterial pressure
   c. Peak arterial pressure
   d. Central venous pressure
   e. Mean arterial pressure
4. What percentage of the total blood volume is contained on the venous side of circulation?
   a. 5
   b. 10
   c. 15
   d. 35
   e. 65
5. What percentage of blood volume can be lost before a significant decrease in blood pressure is noted?
   a. 10
   b. 20
   c. 30
   d. 40
   e. 50
6. The first indicator of a compensatory mechanism responding to lost blood volume is
   a. decreased systolic pressure.
   b. decreased diastolic pressure.
   c. reduced skin perfusion.
   d. increased mean arterial pressure.
   e. reduced mean arterial pressure.
7. An arterial pressure pulsation is
   i.   not immediately transmitted to the periphery.
   ii. generated outward in a wave moving faster and faster.
   iii. up to 100 times the speed of actual blood flow.
   iv. felt long before blood reaches the point of palpation.
   v.   also backward movement toward the heart.

a. i, ii, iii

b. ii, iii, iv

c. iii, iv, v

d. i, iii, v

e. i, ii, iii, iv, v

8. Which of the following organ systems receives the largest percentage of total cardiac output?

a. Liver

b. Kidneys

c. Brain

d. Muscle

e. Skin

9. Pulmonary vascular resistance is approximately _____ times lower than systemic vascular resistance.

a. 1–2

b. 3–4

c. 6–7

d. 10–15

e. 20–30

10. Critical closing pressure of an artery describes

a. the collapse of a vessel when muscle tone overcomes blood pressure.

b. the pressure required to close the pulmonic valves.

c. the pressure required to close the aortic valves.

d. the pressure required to close the heart valves.

e. the pressure needed to open both the pulmonic and aortic valves of the heart.

12

FLUIDS AND ELECTROLYTE BALANCE

OBJECTIVES

1. List the substances involved in the diffusion process and their respective functions.

2. Identify the relative capillary permeability of NaCl, glucose, hemoglobin, myoglobin, and albumin.

Matthews LR: CARDIOPULMONARY ANATOMY AND PHYSIOLOGY. © 1996 Lippincott–Raven Publishers.

3. Differentiate between passive and active transport.

4. Note the significance of electrical forces in the process of diffusion.

5. Set forth the four forces that determine fluid movement through the capillary membrane.

6. Define the term *filtration coefficient.*

7. Discuss the role of the lymphatics in fluid movement out of the interstitial space.

8. Define the term *edema* and enumerate the safety factors that protect against its formation.

9. Review the anatomy of the lymphatics associated with the thorax.

10. Describe the basic process of fluid movement into and through the lymphatics.

11. Discuss the distribution of body fluids in the body.

12. Characterize the movement of water between the plasma and interstitial fluid.

13. Explain the concept of water balance.

14. Describe the concept of effective circulating volume.

15. Provide details on the regulation of circulating blood volume through volume receptors.

16. Reiterate the law of electroneutrality.

17. Describe the basic principles of using intravenous solutions.

18. Identify the normal values for electrolytes in extracellular and intracellular fluid.

19. Demonstrate understanding of the physiological functions of electrolytes.

20. List the effects of hyper- and hypokalemia.

21. Identify the symptoms of hyper- and hypocalcemia.

The body's fluid, which is composed of water, electrolytes, and other bioactive compounds, is classified as either *intracellular* or *extracellular*, depending on whether it is found within the cell compartment or outside the cell.

This chapter concerns itself with these fluids, as well as with the electrolytes found in these fluids. Electrolytes are important because they break down into their ionic components in solution, thus creating a medium through which an electric current can pass. The body's store of electrolytes includes a number of salts, including sodium (Na^+), potassium (K^+), and chlorine (Cl^-). Their role in this conductivity is what allows action potentials to translate into physiological activity.

Electrolyte disturbances and fluid shifts from one body compartment to another can have a dramatic impact on cardiovascular function. It is for this reason that a fundamental understanding of the forces governing fluid movement and electrolyte balance is important in the study of cardiopulmonary care.

▼ FLUIDS AND THEIR CHARACTERISTICS

The movement of fluid in the body occurs between three major fluid compartments:

1. Intracellular
2. Interstitial
3. Intravascular

The dividing membranes between these compartments are the cell membrane and the capillary wall; the interstitium is the medium between the cell mass and the capillary wall.

Diffusion, which involves continuous interchange between the blood and interstitial fluids, is the most important method of moving fluids and substances from one body compartment to another. Because all substances are not created equal, the respiratory therapy student should take into consideration the characteristics of these substances that can influence diffusibility. They are

1. water solubility.
2. lipid solubility.
3. their water content.
4. molecular size.

Water Solubility

Ions and glucose are extremely soluble in water and not at all fat soluble. Therefore, the lipid membrane of endothelial cells is relatively impermeable to ions and glucose. These substances move primarily between the blood and interstitial fluids through capillary pores.

Lipid Solubility

Most gases, including oxygen and carbon dioxide, are lipid soluble. This means that they can diffuse directly through the cell membranes of the capillary. Lipid-soluble substances are much more highly diffusible than are lipid-insoluble substances.

TABLE 12-1 Relative Capillary Permeability to Various Substances	
Substance	Relative Capillary Permeability (compared with water)
NaCl	Approximately equal, decreased by 4%
Glucose	40% less permeable
Hemoglobin	100 times less permeable
Myoglobin	30 times less permeable
Albumin	10,000 times less permeable

Water

Water is second only to lipid-soluble substances in diffusibility. Water diffuses directly through the endothelial wall into the interstitium and then into the cell. It also moves through pores in the capillary membrane.

Molecular Size

Pores in the capillary membrane are about 20 times the size of a water molecule (H_2O). Plasma proteins are larger than the opening in the pore. Therefore, the ability of a substance to pass through the pores in the capillary membrane is dependent on its molecular size. (See Table 12-1 for a comparison of how various substances move through the capillary membrane.)

▼ PASSIVE AND ACTIVE TRANSPORT

There are two types of diffusion: active and passive. **Passive diffusion** does not require energy and occurs in response to a pressure gradient. If the diffusion process requires energy, it is referred to as **active transport**. Active transport is necessary for movement of solutes against concentration gradients and/or electrical gradients.

Significance of Electrical Forces

The movement of ions across a membrane is affected by the electrical potential across the membrane. Positively charged particles are attracted to the negative side of the membrane, and negatively charged particles are attracted to its positive side (Figure 12-1).

Active transport is responsible for maintaining the concentration gradient across the cell membrane (Na^+–K^+ pump). A pump responsible for maintaining this gradient is located in the cell membrane. It seems to be regulated by the enzyme adenosine triphosphatase (ATPase). This enzyme converts ATP to adenosine diphosphate (ADP) and in the process releases energy that can be used in the process of active transport.

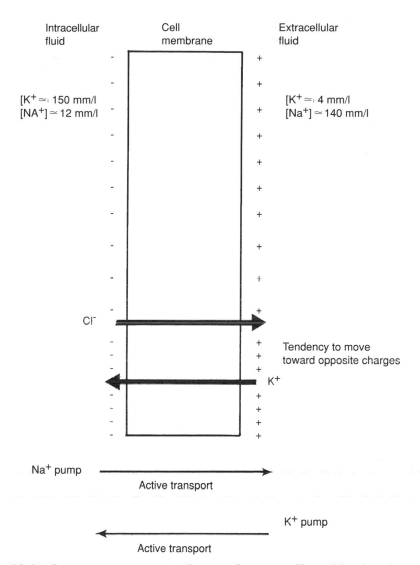

Figure 12-1.   Ion movement across the membrane is effected by the electrical potential across the membrane.

Interstitium

Between 15% and 20% of the body is made up of spaces between cells. This region is referred to as the interstitium and consists of collagen fiber bundles and proteoglycan filaments, which form a mesh of fine reticular filaments. The combination of substances in this area is referred to as "tissue gel." This region also contains free fluid, normally in small quantities. However, if edema develops, the quantity of fluid can increase significantly.

Forces Determining Fluid Movement Through the Capillary Membrane

There are four forces governing the movement of fluid across the capillary membrane:

1. Capillary pressure, a positive pressure generated by the heart's pumping action, has a tendency to push fluid out of the capillary and into the interstitial space (average pressure approximately 20 mmHg).
2. Interstitial fluid pressure is thought to be a negative pressure (2–7 mmHg subatmospheric) and therefore has a tendency to pull fluid back into the interstitium.
3. Plasma colloid osmotic pressure has a tendency to pull fluid into the vascular space (albumin).
4. Interstitial colloid osmotic pressure has a tendency to pull fluid out of the vascular space.

Figure 12-2 is a schematic representation of normal fluid movement across a capillary membrane. The regulation and stability of the movement of body fluids depend on an appropriate balance between these forces.

The forces affecting fluid movement change as the blood moves from the arterial to the venous end of the capillary bed. A small quantity of fluid exits

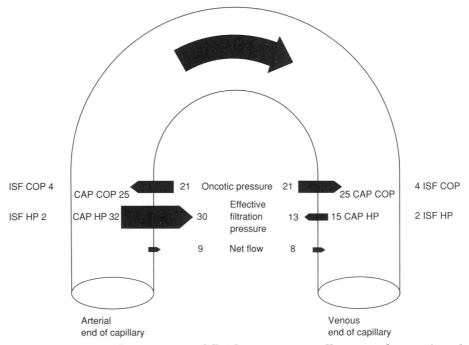

Figure 12-2.   Normal movement of fluids across a capillary membrane. (Porth, C.M., Pathophysiology: Concepts of Altered Health States, 4th ed. Philadelphia: J.B. Lippincott, 1994, with permission.)

the vasculature at the arterial end of the capillary bed and reenters at the venous end. The net outward movement at the arterial end is approximately 9 mmHg; at the venous end it has a net inward force of approximately 8 mmHg. This difference is directly related to the variation in blood pressure (capillary pressure). Blood pressure is the primary force pushing fluid out of the capillary bed, and as it decreases, the force moving outward decreases. When all forces are compared, a slight imbalance exists in favor of fluid moving into the interstitial spaces. This fluid is picked up by the lymphatics and returned to the bloodstream.

Filtration Coefficient

This is a term used to describe the filtration rate in terms of pressure generated to filter fluid out of the capillaries. It is therefore expressed in milliliters of fluid per minute per mmHg. It can be used to predict variations in fluid movement characteristic of various physiological anomalies.

▼ LYMPHATICS

The lymphatics can move excess fluid out of the interstitial space and, more importantly, they can remove large particles such as bacteria, nutrients, fats, and protein from the fluid. The majority of lymph flows into the thoracic duct and into the venous system at the junction of the left internal jugular vein and the subclavian vein (Figure 12-3). The remainder enters venous circulation via the right lymph duct at the junction of the right subclavian vein and internal jugular vein.

Only about 10% of the fluid enters the lymphatics and returns to venous circulation; the rest is reabsorbed into the venous capillary bed (Figure 12-4). Total lymphatic flow returning from the body is approximately 120 mL/hour. An increase in interstitial pressure from edema can increase lymph flow to 50 times its normal rate. This may be a result of

1. increased capillary pressure.
2. decreased plasma colloidal osmotic pressure.
3. increased interstitial fluid protein (increasing osmotic pressure).
4. increased capillary permeability.

▼ EDEMA

Edema is defined as the presence of excess fluid in the interstitium. Generally, extra fluid moving into the interstitium is simply removed by the lymphatics.

As long as the interstitial pressure remains negative, increased interstitial pressure does not have a significant impact on the volume of accumulating fluid. However, once the interstitial pressure becomes positive, the volume

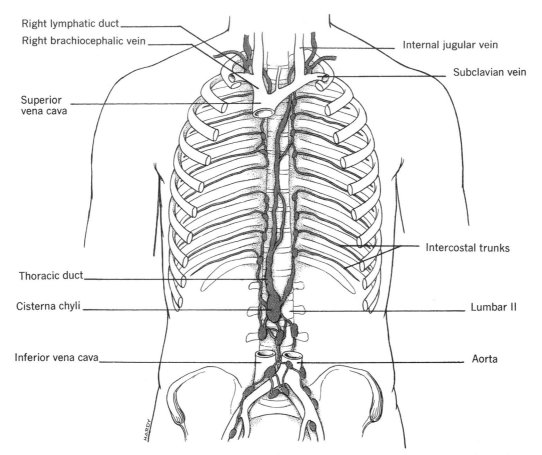

Right lymphatic duct

Right brachiocephalic vein

Internal jugular vein

Subclavian vein

Superior
vena cava

Intercostal trunks

Thoracic duct

Cisterna chyli

Lumbar II

Inferior vena cava

Aorta

Figure 12-3.   The lymphatics. (Chaffee, E.E. and Lytle, I.M., Basic Physiology and Anatomy, 4th ed. Philadelphia: J.B. Lippincott, 1980, with permission.)

of fluid accumulating increases exponentially, even with a small increase in pressure. This results in a clinically significant formation of edema.

Safety Factors that Protect Against the Formation of Edema

Under normal circumstances fluid is kept from building up in tissues by the operation of several distinct mechanisms: negative interstitial pressure, adequate lymph drainage, and reduced colloid osmotic pressure.

The negative pressure of the interstitial space is -5 mmHg. It has already been stated that as long as pressure remains negative, a significant volume accumulation will not occur. Therefore, this gives us a safety margin of -5 mmHg.

Lymph drainage also provides a safety against fluid accumulation. It has been estimated that this safety is equivalent to 5 mmHg.

When lymph flow is increased, proteins are washed out with the fluid.

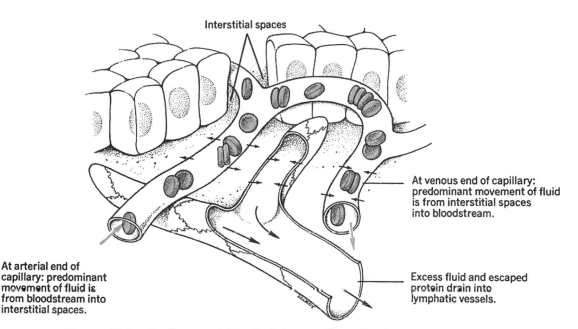

Interstitial spaces

At venous end of capillary: predominant movement of fluid is from interstitial spaces into bloodstream.

At arterial end of capillary: predominant movement of fluid is from bloodstream into interstitial spaces.

Excess fluid and escaped protein drain into lymphatic vessels.

Figure 12-4.   At the arterial end of the capillary, fluid moves primarily from the bloodstream into the interstitial spaces. At the venous end, fluid generally moves from the interstitial spaces into the bloodstream. (Chaffee, E.E. and Lytle, I.M., Basic Physiology and Anatomy, 4th ed. Philadelphia: J.B. Lippincott, 1980, with permission.)

This decreases the colloid osmotic pressure of the interstitial fluid and can add another 5 mmHg to the safety factor.

When adding all three factors together, a total safety of 15 mmHg is realized. In essence, this means that the capillary pressure can increase as much as 15 mmHg above its normal value before edema makes a clinical appearance; likewise, capillary osmotic pressure can decrease by 15 mmHg below its normal value before significant edema occurs.

The same principles apply in the lung as in systemic circulation. However, in the lung, low capillary pressure increases the normal safety factor to approximately 20 mmHg.

▼ DISTRIBUTION OF BODY FLUIDS

Total body water (TBW) accounts for approximately 50% of total body weight in females and 60% in males, and it is distributed as noted in Table 12-2.

Water Movement Between the Cell and Extracellular Fluids

Osmotic forces determine the distribution of water in the various body compartments. Na^+ salts provide the primary extracellular osmotic force and hold

TABLE 12-2   Distribution of Total Body Water
50% in muscle
20% in skin
10% in blood
20% in other organ systems

water within the extracellular space. K^+ salts provide the primary intracellular osmotic force and hold water in the cells. Even though the cell membrane is permeable to Na^+ and K^+, the Na^+–K^+ pump in the cell membrane keeps the electrolytes in their respective compartments. The volumes of extracellular and intracellular water depend on TBW and the ratio of exchangeable Na^+ to exchangeable K^+.

Water Movement Between the Plasma and Interstitial Fluid

The capillary membrane is semipermeable to Na^+ salts and glucose. This means that the interstitium does not have its own substances to create an osmotic pressure. In contrast, plasma proteins cannot cross the membrane easily, meaning they provide an effective osmotic force. The plasma proteins act to pull water out of the interstitium and into the vascular space. The pressure created by plasma protein is called **colloid osmotic pressure**.

As described earlier, fluid is kept from moving rapidly into the capillary or out into the vascular space by counterbalancing pressures.

Water Balance

Despite a wide range of daily variations in fluid intake, the volume and composition of body fluids is kept within an extremely narrow range. Excretion is adjusted to match intake to keep this balance in check. Excess intake can be easily dealt with by increasing fluid output through urination, defecation, and/or vaporization from the skin and respiratory tract. Urinary water loss through the kidneys is highly variable, depending on the hypothalamic hormone antidiuretic hormone (ADH). This hormone reduces urinary water loss. A thirst mechanism is responsible for stimulating the desire for water intake.

Reduced fluid input is more difficult to deal with. This situation can only be corrected by increasing input from one of three sources:

1. Drinking
2. Food containing water
3. Water generated by the oxidation of carbohydrates, fats, and proteins during their metabolism

▼ REGULATION OF EFFECTIVE CIRCULATING VOLUME

Normal tissue perfusion is achieved through the regulation of cardiac output, vascular resistance, and the excretion of Na^+ and water. Extracellular volume is composed of circulating volume and interstitial volume:

$$\text{Extracellular volume} = \text{circulating volume} + \text{interstitial volume}$$

Extracellular fluid (ECF) volume is dependent on its concentration of sodium (Na^+), and circulating volume varies directly with extracellular fluid volume. Regulating serum sodium concentration regulates circulating blood volume.

We are concerned with effective circulating blood volume because it is the volume of blood that comes in contact with the capillary bed for effective exchange of gases and nutrients. Blood that bypasses the capillary circulation through an arteriovenous fistula (**shunt**) is not effectively exchanged in the capillary bed. This shunted blood is referred to as **ineffective circulating volume**; it is arterial blood entering venous circulation.

In the absence of arteriovenous fistula (left-to-right shunt), the relationship between extracellular volume and effective circulating volume can still be significantly disturbed by a number of clinical abnormalities. Hepatic cirrhosis, for example, may result in a fluid accumulation in the peritoneal space (ascites). Infection in the pleura can result in a pleural effusion. Both cases can reduce circulating volume but not extracellular volume. Internal hemorrhage can have a dramatic impact on effective circulating volume, resulting in both blood cell and fluid loss, a possibly life-threatening situation.

Regulating Sodium and Effective Circulating Volume

The kidneys are responsible for regulating plasma sodium concentrations and, therefore, water volume. If sodium ions are retained, water is retained; if sodium ions are excreted, water is excreted. A high sodium concentration (from intake) elevates plasma osmolality to stimulate both thirst and the secretion of ADH to reduce water output by the kidneys. This increases effective circulating volume.

Regulation Through Volume Receptors

The kidney and extrarenal circulation can sense circulating volume changes. Macula densa cells in the distal tubule of the kidney and stretch receptors in the afferent arterioles impact on the renin-angiotensin-aldosterone system. There are also volume receptors in the left atrium and pressure receptors in the carotid sinuses. These receptors impact on ADH release to regulate circulating blood volume.

The sympathetic nervous system too has a regulatory effect on circulating volume. Pressure receptors in the carotid sinuses, aortic arch, left atrium, and large pulmonary veins provide feedback for regulation of cardiac output, vascular resistance, and tubular sodium reabsorption. If hypotension is sensed, cardiac output increases, vascular resistance increases, and sodium is retained by the kidneys. This is all in an attempt to maintain adequate perfusion to the tissues.

The combination of all of these compensatory mechanisms results in a continuous attempt to return effective circulating volume to normal.

▼ LAW OF ELECTRONEUTRALITY

In a given body compartment the total number of cations (positive ions) must be equal to the total number of anions (negative ions). If an anion or a cation is lost from a body compartment, it must be replaced or balanced.

For example, there is an inverse relationship between HCO_3^- and Cl^-. If the total number of ions is constant and the HCO_3^- concentration increases, Cl^- concentration decreases (hypochloremia). If Cl^- is lost, then the HCO_3^- increases correspondingly.

If hypokalemia develops, K^+ (potassium ion) leaves the cell because of the resulting concentration gradient. To maintain electroneutrality, H^+ (hydrogen ion) and Na^+ (sodium ion) enter the cell. The H^+ causes an intracellular acidosis. This intracellular acidosis causes the kidney to secrete H^+ and retain HCO_3^-.

Conversely, acidosis (increased $[H^+]$) causes K^+ to leave the cell and alkalosis (decreased $[H^+]$) causes K^+ to enter the cell. The kidney responds by increasing the excretion of K^+ in alkalosis and decreasing excretion of K^+ during acidosis.

▼ INTRAVENOUS SOLUTIONS

There are a vast number of intravenous solutions available for use in various clinical situations. These solutions and the basic principles for their use are as follows.

Dextrose Solution

Glucose is quickly metabolized to carbon dioxide and water. This makes glucose administration physiologically equivalent to administering pure water. It can be most effectively used to provide replacement of water due to insensible loss or to correct hypernatremia (excess of sodium in the blood) resulting from a water deficiency.

Saline (NaCl) Solution

Generally, hypovolemic patients are deficient in sodium and water. Either vomiting or diarrhea can result in this form of hypovolemia. Isotonic, hypotonic, and hypertonic saline solutions can be used. *Isotonic* saline has the same sodium concentration as plasma (0.9%). *Hypotonic* saline has a lower concentration of sodium than does saline and, of course, *hypertonic* saline has a higher concentration of sodium than does plasma. Isotonic or hypertonic solutions should be used to replace water when the patient has a deficiency of water and sodium (hyponatremia). Conversely, hypotonic solutions should be used when the patient is hypovolemic with hypernatremia, in the same way dextrose and water is used.

Saline (NaCl) and Dextrose Solutions

A combination of saline and dextrose in a solution can be used in a fashion similar to how each is used alone. These solutions have the added benefit of providing the body with needed calories in the form of glucose.

Ringer's Lactate

This solution contains physiological concentrations of K^+, Ca^{++}, Na^+, and Cl^-. It also contains lactate, which is quickly metabolized into HCO_3^- once it is in the body. Although this is an attempt to provide a physiological solution, there is little evidence that it has advantages over other isotonic solutions.

Plasma Volume Expanders

When Na^+ is administered intravenously, it freely diffuses across the capillary membrane. This results in expansion of both the intravascular and interstitial volumes. When water or isotonic solutions are administered, intracellular volume also increases. The water is distributed between all three compartments. Therefore, dextrose in water expands ECF 33% less than an equivalent volume of isotonic solution.

In contrast to this, the administration of albumin directly expands intravascular volume. Albumin increases the plasma oncotic pressure and draws several times its volume of fluid into the vascular space from the interstitium. This may be necessary with hypovolemic shock or with hypoalbuminemia.

▼ ELECTROLYTES

Electrolytes are essential for normal physiological functions. They serve a variety of functions, including

1. maintenance of electroneutrality in the body.
2. maintenance of osmotic equilibrium between ECF and intracellular fluid (ICF).
3. regulation of neuromuscular activity.
4. maintenance of ideal conditions for various chemical reactions in the body.

Sodium

About 25% of sodium in the body is nonexchangeable and is found primarily in bone. The exchangeable sodium is found primarily in ECF with the remainder in ICF. Sodium accounts for about 90% of all cations in ECF. Although the kidneys play the major role in sodium balance, a small amount of this element is put out of the body in feces and sweat.

As described earlier, sodium and its most abundant anion, chloride, are major factors in the loss or retention of water.

Hyponatremia, the depletion of sodium in the plasma, is most commonly associated with actual sodium loss rather than a decrease in intake. Diarrhea can result in the loss of large amounts of sodium-rich water. Sweating also can result in sodium loss, but it is much less common. Reduced aldosterone or osmotic diuretics may cause significant sodium loss. A decreased cardiac output, reduced systemic blood pressure, and reduced skin elasticity are all signs of reduced body fluids reflective of decreased sodium concentrations in ECF. In severe cases, hyponatremia results in

1. acidosis (decreased pH).
2. muscle weakness.
3. decreased muscle reflex, weakness.
4. disorientation.
5. apathy, lethargy.

Hypernatremia often manifests itself as edema. The most common reason is renal failure to excrete sodium. It results in

1. increased reflex activity.
2. increased body temperature.
3. mental impairment.
4. irritability.

Potassium

Potassium is an essential, intracellular ion. Its regulation is vital to normal neuromuscular function. Potassium, like sodium, is excreted in sweat, feces, and urine. The kidneys play the primary role in regulating its excretion.

Reduced potassium develops when there is a net loss of potassium from the cells. However, reduced plasma potassium can occur when potassium shifts from ECF to ICF (hypokalemia). A decreased intake can cause a mild deficiency, although severe depletion results from abnormal losses rather than decreased intake. Loss of potassium may result when excessive potassium is released from cells, as in trauma, or the kidneys excrete an overabundance, as in the use of some diuretics.

Tissue Trauma

When cells are destroyed, potassium is released into the plasma, causing transient hyperkalemia. Partially resulting from the influence of aldosterone, the kidneys respond by excreting the excessive plasma potassium. The result is a decreased total body potassium with a normal or even elevated plasma concentration. The normal response to potassium depletion is

1. cardiac dysrhythmias.
2. weak skeletal muscles.
3. alkalosis (or increased pH).
4. fatigue.
5. confusion.
6. electrocardiogram showing a flat or inverted T-wave.

Potassium excess (hyperkalemia) may result in a toxic state and cardiac arrest. If aldosterone levels decrease or acute renal failure develops, adequate amounts of potassium may not be excreted and serious hyperkalemia may result. A plasma potassium concentration above 7–13 mmol/L is usually lethal. Milder cases may result in a metabolic acidosis as hydrogen ion exchanges with potassium.

Calcium

The vast majority (99%) of calcium is deposited in bone as crystalline salts, composed primarily of calcium and phosphorous. The remaining 1% is in the plasma, ICF, and soft tissues. The physiological significance of calcium results from its concentration in plasma. Approximately one half of the calcium is in its ionized form; the remainder is bound primarily to protein.

Calcium and phosphorous are necessary for bone formation. Calcium is also a necessary cofactor in blood clotting and is essential to muscle function.

Hypocalcemia may result in tetany, which can rapidly result in death. Hypercalcemia results in depression of muscle contractility and skeletal muscle weakness.

Phosphorous

Phosphorous is an extremely important mineral. It is essential for the production of the high-energy phosphate compounds (such as ATP and ADP) and is also necessary for bone formatiom.

Magnesium

Found primarily in muscle and bone, a reduction in magnesium may result in hyper-irritability and convulsions.

▼ CONCLUSION

Fluid and electrolyte balance is essential to normal cardiac and skeletal muscle function. Because the heart is responsible for oxygen delivery to the tissues and skeletal muscles provide the forces needed to breathe, close monitoring of both fluid and electrolyte levels is important.

❖ Review Questions

1. Which of the following forces govern the movement of fluid across the capillary membrane?
   i. Capillary pressure
   ii. Interstitial pressure
   iii. Plasma colloid osmotic pressure
   iv. Interstitial colloid osmotic pressure

   a. i, ii, iii
   b. ii, iii, iv
   c. iii, iv
   d. i, iii
   e. All of the above

2. Total lymphatic flow returning from the body is approximately (mL/hr)
   a. 10.
   b. 50.
   c. 70.
   d. 120.
   e. 500.

3. An increase in interstitial pressure from edema can increase lymph flow to _____ times its normal rate.
   a. 10
   b. 20
   c. 50
   d. 100
   e. 210

4. The total gain and loss of body water in an adult per day is approximately (in liters)
   a. 0.5.
   b. 1.0.
   c. 2.5.
   d. 4.5.
   e. 5.0.

5. Which of the following may play a role in regulation of circulating blood volume?
   i. Macula densa cells
   ii. Afferent arterial stretch receptors
   iii. Left atrial volume receptors
   iv. Carotid sinus pressure receptors
   v. ADH

   a. i, ii, iii

    b. ii, iii, iv

    c. iii, iv, v

    d. i, iii, v

    e. All of the above

6. The normal response to hypokalemia is

    i. alkalosis.

    ii. fatigue.

    ii. confusion.

    iv. flat or inverted T wave on ECG.

    v. prolonged P-R interval.

    a. i, ii, iii

    b. ii, iii, iv

    c. iii, iv, v

    d. i, ii, iii, iv

    c. All of the above

13

ACID–BASE BALANCE

OBJECTIVES

1. Define pH.
2. Differentiate between acids and bases.
3. Describe the Henderson-Hasselbalch equation.
4. Explain the concept of buffers.
5. List four methods of dealing with H^+ loading and/or unloading.
6. Discuss the mechanism of HCO_3 retrieval by the kidney tubular cells.
7. Outline the exchange mechanism in the kidneys that is responsible for H^+ buffering.
8. Identify the renal mechanisms responsible for dealing with metabolic acids.
9. Describe the secretion function and metabolism of aldosterone.
10. Characterize antidiuretic hormone.

Matthews LR: CARDIOPULMONARY ANATOMY AND PHYSIOLOGY. © 1996 Lippincott–Raven Publishers.

Normal metabolism results in the production of hydrogen ions, the normal extracellular hydrogen ion concentration $[H^+]$ of which is approximately 0.00000004 moles, or equivalents (eq), per liter. This is close to one millionth of the "per liter" concentration of Na^+, K^+, Cl^-, and HCO_3^-. However, its regulation within a narrow range is essential for normal cellular function. Primarily because of its high level of reactivity with protein, hydrogen ion can interact with proteins and alter function. For example, the rate of glycolysis (enzymatic hydrolysis in the body) is inversely related to the presence of hydrogen ions or hydrogen ion concentration $[H^+]$.

In the body, hydrogen ions are hydrated or combined with water. In this state they are referred to as hydronium ions. Because this is not of clinical significance, we will confine our discussion to hydrogen ion as an independent ion. The term *hydrogen ion concentration* $[H^+]$ can be used to identify the presence of hydrogen in a given body compartment. However, if we try to express hydrogen ion concentration in moles per liter, the numbers are extremely small and cumbersome. For this reason, the term pH (potential for hydrogen) is used to describe the concentration of hydrogen ion in a given compartment of the body.

▼ DEFINITION OF pH

The definition of pH is the negative log of $[H^+]$.

$$pH = -\log [H^+]$$

Because the logarithm would be a negative number, when we express the concentration of H^+ as the negative log, it becomes a positive number, thus making it easier to use.

▼ ACIDS AND BASES

Acids are substances that can donate H^+, and bases are substances that can accept H^+. Table 13-1 lists the pH and dissociated versions of common compounds. Note that the acid produces a H^+. This contributes to the amount of

TABLE 13-1 pH and Dissociated Versions of Common Compounds	
Acid	**Base**
H_2CO_3	$H^+ + HCO_3^-$
HCl	$H^+ + Cl^-$
NH_4^+	$H^+ + NH_3^-$
H_2PO_4	$H^+ + HPO_4^{2-}$

available H^+ in solution. The reaction occurs in both directions: the H^+ can combine with base and take the H^+ out of solution into its combined form.

The vast majority of acid is actually excreted by the lungs in the form of carbon dioxide (CO_2). If for some reason CO_2 is not expelled by the lungs, H^+ will begin to build up. Carbon dioxide itself is neither acid nor base, but it combines with water to produce carbonic acid in the following manner:

$$CO_2 + H_2O \ H_2CO_3 \ H_+ + HCO_3^-$$

There are a handful of acids that do not produce carbonic acid. These are primarily produced by the metabolism of proteins. For example, sulfur-containing amino acids are oxidized into sulfuric acid (H_2SO_4). These H^+ ions are excreted by the kidneys.

Metabolism of carbohydrate and fat normally generates approximately 13,000 mmol of carbonic acid per day, which is removed from the body via the lung in the form of CO_2. The kidneys excrete approximately 60 mmol/day of acid. Ventilatory failure would result in a toxic build-up of hydrogen ions within a matter of minutes. On the other hand, it could take days for a toxic hydrogen ion build-up to occur as the result of kidney failure.

▼ HENDERSON-HASSELBALCH EQUATION

Acids and bases are continually being added to and removed from extracellular fluid. The delicate balance between acids and bases in the blood, which must be maintained, is described by the Henderson-Hasselbalch equation:

$$pH = pKa + log[HCO_3^-] \ base/[H_2CO_3] \ acid$$
$$pH = 6.1 + 1.3$$
$$= 7.4$$

pKa is the dissociation constant for carbonic acid. It is expressed as the negative log of the dissociation constant and its value is 6.1. This means that at a pH of 6.1, 50% of the carbonic acid would be dissociated and 50% would not be dissociated.

When this value is added to the relationship between acid and base, the number of available hydrogen ions is expressed in terms of pH. The normal relationship between base and acid is 20:1, and the log of 20 is 1.3.

A pH of 7.4 is the mean value for plasma. The normal pH in humans is 7.35–7.45. It can be seen that if the relationship between acid and base were to change, so would the pH.

As the concentration of hydrogen ions increases, the pH decreases and vice versa. The reason for this stems from the fact that pH is actually a negative number. Therefore, a larger negative number actually is indicative of a lower concentration of hydrogen ions. It is important to remember that pH and hy-

TABLE 13-2 pH for Acidosis and Alkalosis		
[H$^+$] and pH	Acidosis	pH <7.35
[H$^+$] and [H]	Alkalosis	pH > 7.45

drogen ion concentration are inversely related. Table 13-2 outlines the relationship between numerical pH and **alkalosis** (excess alkalinity) and **acidosis** (increased acidity).

When pH is measured and reported, it is extracellular, or plasma, pH we are considering. In a number of body tissues, the intracellular pH is actually lower, or more acidic, than extracellular pH. Regardless of this fact, plasma pH directly reflects intracellular pH, with the added advantage that it is much easier to measure.

▼ BUFFERS

Large changes in hydrogen ion concentration are prevented by buffers, mechanisms that accept or release hydrogen ions. In actuality, the body's buffers are primarily weak acids that can take up or release hydrogen ions, thus minimizing any major swings in hydrogen ion concentration.

For example,

$$H_2CO_3 \; H^+ \; + \; HCO_3^-$$

If hydrogen ions are added to extracellular fluid, they will combine with bicarbonate (HCO_3^-) to form carbonic acid (H_2CO_3). The reverse also will occur. If hydrogen ions are lost from extracellular fluid, the reaction will reverse and H_2CO_3 will release its H^+ into solution.

▼ REGULATION OF ACID-BASE BALANCE

There are four methods of dealing with H^+ loading and/or unloading, processes by which ions are, respectively, introduced into or removed from a system:

1. Extracellular buffering by bicarbonate (HCO_3^-)
2. Intracellular buffering
3. Ventilatory buffering
4. Renal regulation of H^+

Extracellular Buffers

HCO_3^- is the most important extracellular buffer. It is an effective buffer for noncarbonic acids but not for carbonic acid, which is buffered by intracellular buffers. Plasma phosphates and proteins also function as buffers but to a lesser degree.

HCO_3^-/CO_2 Buffer System

Under normal circumstances, approximately 95% of all acid produced during metabolism is in the form of CO_2. Therefore, the HCO_3^-/CO_2 buffer system is very important.

Approximately 200 mL of carbon dioxide is produced in the body every minute. This carbon dioxide must enter the bloodstream and be transported to the lungs, where it is exhaled. The following reaction occurs:

$$CO_2 + H_2O \; H_2CO_3 \; H^+ + HCO_3^-$$

Remember, the solubility coefficient for CO_2 in plasma is 0.03 mmol/L/mmHg/37°. When the $PaCO_2$ is 40 mmHg, the amount of CO_2 dissolved in the plasma is expressed as

$$40 \text{ mmHg} \times 0.03 = 1.2 \text{ mmol/L}$$

The hydration of CO_2 in plasma is slow. In plasma, there are about 500 molecules of CO_2 for every molecule of H_2CO_3. But there is a direct relationship between the amount of carbon dioxide in plasma and the amount of carbonic acid. The presence of carbonic anhydrase in the red blood cell (RBC) and the renal tubular cells makes this reaction occur much more rapidly because carbonic anhydrase catalyzes the reaction.

Intracellular Buffers

In the cell, proteins, phosphates, and, most importantly, hemoglobin (which resides in RBCs) act as buffers:

$$H^+ + Hb^- \rightleftharpoons HHb$$

When carbon dioxide is buffered inside the RBC, the hydrogen ion combines with the hemoglobin molecule and HCO_3^- diffuses out of the cell, exchanging with Cl^- to maintain the cell's electroneutrality.

When a hydrogen ion moves into a cell from the plasma, Na^+ and K^+ move out of the cell into the plasma to maintain electroneutrality. This can result in a dangerous increase in plasma K^+ concentration. Acidosis results in hyperkalemia because as plasma H^+ concentration is reduced, plasma K^+ concentration decreases. Na^+ does not become a problem in this process because the high plasma concentration of Na^+ is simply not changed enough to make a clinically significant difference.

Bone as Buffer

There is a large store of carbonate (CO_3^{-2}) in bone, which plays a role in buffering acid and base loads in the body. A significant amount of buffering occurs in the bone when there is an acute change in acid or base.

Buffering Through Ventilation

Under normal circumstances, the exhalation of CO_2 from the lungs derives from the following reaction:

$$CO_2 + H_2O \: H_2CO_3 \: H^+ + HCO_3^-$$

An increase in alveolar ventilation removes more H^+ by shifting this reaction.

Hydrogen ion added to the blood (metabolic acidosis) can increase ventilation as much as sixfold. The response of the respiratory system can turn a potentially life-threatening acidosis into a clinical problem that is much less threatening. Although the response may appear immediately, the maximum response may take up to 24 hours to manifest itself. The important thing to remember here is that increasing ventilation removes more CO_2 and hence H^+. Conversely, decreased ventilation removes less CO_2 and hence less H^+. Hydrogen ion stimulates ventilation to facilitate greater removal of CO_2 and vice versa.

Renal Regulation of H^+

The kidneys play a role in acid–base balance by

1. regulating HCO_3^- loss in the urine (reabsorbing or excreting).
2. excreting H^+ (up to 100 mmol/day).

Together, these two processes remove only 5% of the total amount of acid from the body every day. The importance of these mechanisms stems from the fact that

1. HCO_3^- cannot be reabsorbed or excreted through the lungs.
2. nonvolatile acids can only be removed through the kidneys.

The kidneys cannot excrete significant quantities of free hydrogen ions. These hydrogen ions must be combined with urinary buffers and then converted to NH_3 and then again to NH_4^+. The phosphate and ammonia buffer systems are the most important buffer systems for removing excess hydrogen ions through the urine. Urate and citrate are less important buffers, but they too can remove excess hydrogen ions from the body.

Phosphate as a Urine Buffer

Phosphate becomes an important buffer in the tubular fluid of the kidney. It exists as both HPO_4^{-2} and $H_2PO_4^-$ in relatively high concentrations. This is because it is poorly reabsorbed into the body, and as water is removed from the tubular fluid, the concentration of phosphate increases. This mechanism removes H^+ by converting HPO_4^{-2} to H_2PO_4 and in doing so removing a H^+. Each time a H^+ is removed from the plasma, a HCO_3^- is added.

Ammonia as a Urine Buffer

This buffer provides a number of functions. Epithelial cells in the tubules and the thin region of the loop of Henle (the U-shaped portion of a renal tubule) continuously synthesize ammonia from glutamine, which diffuses into the tubular fluid. The ammonia reacts with H^+ to form ammonium ions (NH_3 is converted to NH_4^+). This can be excreted in the urine as it combines with chloride to form ammonium chloride, a weak acid that easily remains in the urine for excretion from the body. In chronic acidosis, this mechanism becomes even more important. When renal tubular cells are in an acidic environment, they produce more ammonia, possibly as much as 10 times the normal quantity. This dramatically enhances the ability to remove H^+ from the urine. Ammonia is lipid soluble and diffuses into the tubular fluid easily. Once it becomes ammonium in ionic form, it is water soluble and remains in the tubular fluid to be removed.

HCO_3^- Retrieval Mechanism

This mechanism is illustrated in Figure 13-1 in three steps:

1. The diffusion of CO_2 into the renal tubular cell from plasma. Once inside the renal tubular cell, the presence of carbonic anhydrase (CA) catalyzes the reaction with water to produce H_2CO_3 and then $H^+ + HCO_3^-$. Without the presence of CA, the reaction would not occur fast enough for this process to be effective.
2. The HCO_3^- returns to the plasma and extracellular fluid in general. Remember, the relationship between base (HCO_3^-) and H_2CO_3 carbonic acid in the blood is 20:1 for a normal pH of 7.4. Therefore, HCO_3 must continuously be retained in the body as H^+ is being excreted. For the HCO_3 to be retained, the H^+ must somehow be removed. The H^+ can be removed by a number of mechanisms: the two primary buffers are phosphate and ammonia. When H^+ diffuses into the tubular fluid it combines with either phosphate to convert to its monobasic form (in which it has one hydrogen atom, which can be replaced by a metal or a positive radical), or it combines with ammonia to form ammonium.
3. Once NH_4^+ and HPO_4^- are formed, they can be removed in the urine. To maintain electroneutrality, Na^+ enters the renal tubular cells as H^+ exits and is then actively transported out into the plasma.

Significance

The renal mechanism is slow in comparison with the respiratory system. It takes hours or days to compensate for an acid–base disturbance. However, it brings the pH back to complete compensation. It functions continuously until the pH is brought back to the normal value (7.35–7.45). It does not gradually decrease in effectiveness as the pH approaches normal, the way the respiratory system does.

The kidneys are also responsible for removing substances formed as the

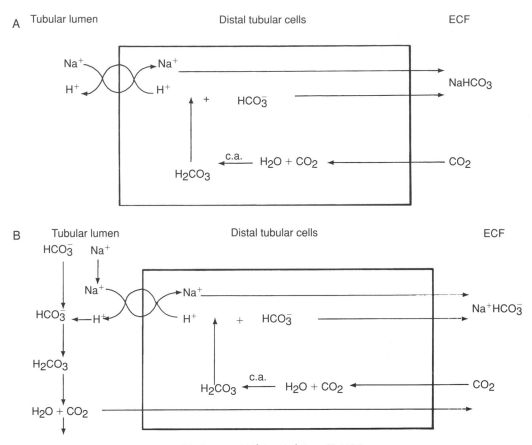

Figure 13-1. **(a) HCO$_3^-$ retrieval by the kidney tubular cells. Using this proposed mechanism, CO$_2$ diffuses into the cell from the bloodstream. In the presence of carbonic anhydrase, CO$_2$ combines with water to form H$_2$CO$_3$. The H$_2$CO$_3$ then ionizes H$^+$ and HCO$_3$. The H$^+$ ions are secreted into the tubular fluid in exchange for Na$^+$. (b) Buffered by NaHCO$_3$. (c) Buffered by Na$_2$HPO$_4$. (d) Buffered by NH$_3$. (Chaffee, E.E. and Lytle, I.M., Basic Physiology and Anatomy, 4th ed. Philadelphia: J.B. Lippincott, 1980, with permission.)**

end product of metabolism such as urea, creatinine, uric acid, and urates. Urea is synthesized in the liver as a method of removing ammonia, a metabolite resulting from the need to produce energy for metabolic purposes. Creatinine is a normal product of skeletal muscle metabolism and is produced at a relatively constant rate. It is not reabsorbed, synthesized, or metabolized by the kidney. Therefore, its removal rate by the kidney is a good indication of renal function.

Uric acid is the waste product of purines (produced by nucleoprotein digestion) in the diet and synthesized in the body. Urates are salts of uric acid. The kidneys are responsible for electrolyte exchange and balance as well as removal or retention of water.

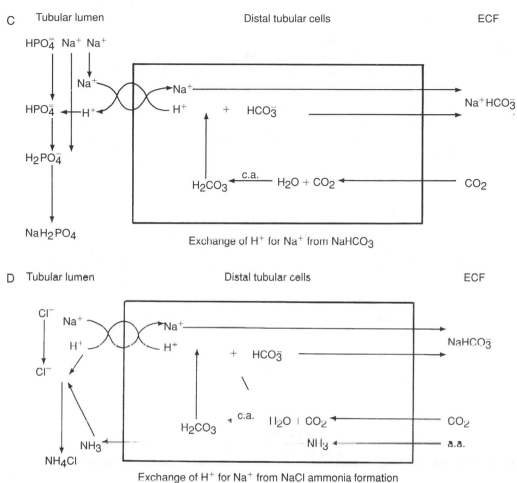

Exchange of H^+ for Na^+ from $NaHCO_3$

Exchange of H^+ for Na^+ from NaCl ammonia formation

Figure 13-1.   Continued

▼ RENAL MECHANISMS

Generally, the kidneys cleanse the blood of unwanted substances. This is accomplished in a number of ways.

Urine pH

The kidney can remove up to 500 mmol/day of either acid or base. If acids are being produced, the urine pH may decrease to as low as 4.5 and when alkali must be removed, the pH may increase to as high as 8.0. Normal urine pH is approximately 6.0 because the body requires a continuous removal of acid under normal metabolic circumstances.

Urine Output

The normal urinary output is variable, depending on the needs of the body and water intake, but an average male puts out approximately 1.5 L/day. This can be increased to as much as 20 L/day if the need should arise.

Aldosterone

This hormone is synthesized in the adrenal cortex (suprarenal glands). It is metabolized in the liver and, to a lesser degree, in the kidney.

Aldosterone increases the reabsorption of Na^+ and secretion of K^+ and H^+. There is a normal quantity of circulating aldosterone. The major stimuli for its secretion are angiotensin II, hyperkalemia, and adrenocorticotropic hormone (ACTH).

If aldosterone levels are elevated (hyperaldosteronism), $NaHCO_3^-$ is reabsorbed and K^+ and H^+ are secreted, resulting in water retention, alkalosis, and hypokalemia. Hyperaldosteronism may result from adrenocortical tumors or Cushing's syndrome.

Antidiuretic Hormone (ADH)

ADH, which may also be called arginine vasopressin, is synthesized in the hypothalamus. After it is produced, it migrates to the pituitary gland, where it is stored, awaiting an appropriate stimulus for release. It is metabolized in both the liver and the kidneys.

The two main stimuli for the release of ADH secretion are

1. increased plasma osmolality.
2. decreased effective circulating volume.

ADH increases renal water reabsorption, leading to conservation of body water. In physiologically stressed patients (i.e., surgical patients), elevated ADH levels may exist for days. Pain afferents may play a role in this reflex response.

▼ CONCLUSION

Because acid–base balance has a profound effect on cardiopulmonary function, the underlying cause of any disturbance in this relationship must be identified as soon as possible so that an appropriate treatment can be instituted. Treatment necessarily focuses on correcting the underlying acidosis or alkalosis, because these conditions can sometimes be life threatening.

❖ Review Questions

1. pH is defined as
   a. $-\log [H^+]$.

    b. [H].

    c. $-\log [H^+] \cdot 6.1$.

    d. $6.1 + [H^+]$.

    e. $[H^+] \pm \log 6.1$.

2. The lung removes approximately _____ mmol of carbonic acid per day.

    a. 60

    b. 120

    c. 500

    d. 7,500

    e. 13,000

3. The kidneys excrete approximately _____ mmol/day of acid.

    a. 60

    b. 120

    c. 500

    d. 7,500

    e. 13,000

4. Normal pH in plasma is

    a. 7.35.

    b. 7.35–7.45.

    c. 7.45.

    d. 7.4.

    e. 7.0–7.5.

5. Which of the following are methods of dealing with H^+ loading and/or unloading?

    i. Extracellular buffering by HCO_3^-

    ii. Intracellular buffering

    iii. Ventilatory buffering

    iv. Sulfatase transferase mechanism

    v. Renal regulation of H^+

    a. i, ii, iii

    b. ii, iii, iv

    c. iii, iv, v

    d. i, ii, iii, v

    e. All of the above

6. A normal K^+ is (in mmol/L)

    a. 3.5–5.0.

    b. 24–32.

    c. 95–105.

    d. 135–145.

    e. 150–157.

14

BLOOD GASES

OBJECTIVES

1. State the normal ranges for arterial and mixed venous blood gases.

2. List the normal ranges for arterial and mixed venous pH.

3. Describe the measured and calculated values of arterial blood gas measurements.

4. Characterize the two major types of acid–base disorders.

5. Discuss the physiological compensation for acid–base disturbances.

Matthews LR: CARDIOPULMONARY ANATOMY AND PHYSIOLOGY. © 1996 Lippincott–Raven Publishers.

6. State the rules of thumb for changing pH.

7. Explain the concept of an anion gap.

8. Discuss the concept of adequate oxygenation.

9. Describe the pulmonary artery catheter.

10. Interpret blood gas values and use in diagnosing underlying disorder.

Information obtained from measuring the PCO_2, PO_2, and pH of arterial blood and mixed venous blood can be extremely helpful when treating respiratory and acid–base disorders. This information, in combination with electrolyte analysis, provides a valuable insight into the many variables encountered in critical care medicine. This chapter will provide a systematic approach to interpretation of blood gases, pH, and electrolyte disturbances.

▼ NORMAL BLOOD GAS VALUES

Our discussion opens with a presentation of normal blood gas values (Table 14-1) and is then enlarged with the subsequent, expanded definitions of those values.

Measured and Calculated Values

Blood gases can be measured directly (as is the case with $PaCO_2$) or calculated from measured values.

TABLE 14-1   Normal Blood Gas Values

Arterial Blood Gases	Mixed Venous Blood Gases	Electrolytes
pH 7.35–7.451	pH 7.33–7.43	Na^+ 135–145
$PaCO_2$ 35–45	$PvCO_2$ 46–481	K^+ 3.5–5.0
PaO_2 80–100	PvO_2 35–45	Cl^- 95–105
Saturation 98%	Saturation 75%	HCO_3^- 24–32
BE ± 2 mmol/L		
Bicarbonate		
Plasma 22–26		
Standard 22–26		
Total CO_2 24–28		

Partial pressure is given in mmHg; bicarbonate and electrolytes are in mmol/L.

Measured Arterial Blood Gases (ABGs)

PaCO₂

This value, defined as the partial pressure of carbon dioxide in arterial blood, is measured in mmHg using a Severinghaus electrode. This apparatus gives a direct moment-to-moment reflection of alveolar ventilation. As alveolar ventilation increases, arterial PCO_2 decreases and vice versa.

PaO₂

Defined as the partial pressure of oxygen in arterial blood, this value is measured in mmHg using a polarographic (Clark) electrode (mmHg). When it decreases to below 50 mmHg, tissue hypoxia is likely. It should be remembered that this value is only a reflection of arterial oxygen content and in a critical care setting should not be relied upon alone.

SaO₂

This value, which indicates the saturation of arterial hemoglobin with oxygen, is measured using a spectrophotometer and is usually expressed as the percentage of oxygen-carrying hemoglobin in arterial blood. It is important that this value be measured and not calculated. It is a much better indicator of arterial oxygen content than PaO_2.

pH

Defined as the negative log of the [H^+] concentration, pH is measured using a Sanz electrode. The hydrogen ion concentration in arterial blood is low at 0.00000004 mmol/L or 4.0×10^{-8} mmol/L. When expressed as the negative logarithm, it converts to 7.40. The normal range is 7.35–7.45. This value is the reciprocal of [H^+]. As pH decreases, [H^+] increases and vice versa. This measurement is a reflection of the balance of acids and bases in the blood.

Calculated Values

Base Excess (BE) or Deficit of Base

Calculated from pH, $PaCO_2$, and hemoglobin concentration, this is an index intended to simplify metabolic contributions to acid–base homeostasis. Negative values indicate a deficit of base; positive values indicate an excess. As with all calculated values, it has limitations and should be considered with caution in a clinical setting. The normal range is ± 2 mmol/L.

Plasma Bicarbonate

Calculated by using the Henderson-Hasselbalch equation, plasma bicarbonate is the index used in an attempt to simplify metabolic contributions to acid–base homeostasis. The normal range is 22–26 mmol/L.

Standard Bicarbonate

This value also uses the Henderson-Hasselbalch equation for calculation. However, in this case, the value is standardized to a PCO_2 of 40 mmHg and a temperature of 37°C. The normal range is 22–26 mmol/L.

Total CO_2

This value is equal to the sum of the plasma bicarbonate and the dissolved CO_2, which is the $PaCO_2$ multiplied by the solubility coefficient of carbon dioxide (0.03 mmol/L/mmHg). This accounts for the increased normal range of 24–28 mmol/L.

Other numerical values can be calculated (i.e., T_{40} standard bicarbonate, BE/deficit of base), but all in an attempt to provide a simple, easy-to-use indication of the metabolic contribution to acid-base homeostasis.

Deciding which calculation is most accurate or convenient is not without controversy. The need to avoid confusion makes it imperative that one choose a value and use it exclusively, even to the point of becoming familiar with its clinical limitations and applications.

Mixed Venous Blood Gases

$P\bar{v}O_2$

The partial pressure of oxygen in mixed venous blood, this value is an indication of the amount of oxygen returning to the heart. It is measured using a polarographic electrode (Clarke). $P\bar{v}O_2$ is reflective of the interaction between the pulmonary and cardiovascular systems. The normal range lies between 35 and 45 mmHg. It is directly related to cardiac output and inversely related to oxygen consumption.

$S\bar{v}O_2$

This value (oxygen saturation in mixed venous blood) can be continuously monitored using a fiberoptic catheter attached to a pulmonary artery catheter. A better indicator of mixed venous oxygenation than $P\bar{v}O_2$, this value can be used as an indicator of cardiovascular and pulmonary effectiveness.

▼ pH BALANCE AND HOMEOSTASIS

The pH range compatible with life is 6.80–7.80. However, as stated earlier, it is normally maintained between 7.35 and 7.45. The balance of acids and bases needed to keep a relatively normal pH is important for normal cellular function. Homeostasis is maintained by

1. pulmonary ventilation and regulation of PCO_2.
2. intra- and extracellular chemical buffering.
3. renal reabsorption and excretion of acid and base.

Disturbances, which are classified as either respiratory or metabolic, can be simple or extremely complex. The four primary acid–base disorders, which will be described in the subsequent two sections, are as follows:

1. Respiratory acidosis
2. Respiratory alkalosis
3. Metabolic acidosis

4. Metabolic alkalosis

Before moving on to dicussions of the above-mentioned disorders, it is worth noting that patients commonly exhibit the mixed abnormalities listed below:

1. Respiratory acidosis combined with metabolic acidosis
2. Respiratory acidosis combined with metabolic alkalosis
3. Metabolic acidosis combined with respiratory alkalosis
4. Metabolic alkalosis combined with respiratory alkalosis

Respiratory Acid–Base Disorder

Respiratory acid–base disorders are characterized by alterations in $PaCO_2$. In hypoventilation, CO_2 levels are above normal and there is resulting acidemia (excessive acidity in the blood). Hyperventilation results in CO_2 levels below normal, with the resulting alkalemia (increased alkalinity of the blood):

$$CO_2 + H_2O \rightleftarrows H_2CO_3 \rightleftarrows HCO_3^- + H^+$$

Hyperventilation   Hypoventilation

Hypoventilation shifts this reaction to the right, increasing available $[H^+]$ (acidosis). Hyperventilation shifts the reaction to the left, decreasing available $[H^+]$ (alkalosis).

Metabolic Acid–Base Disorder

Metabolic disorders are characterized by alterations in the bicarbonate concentration. The kidneys respond to acid–base abnormalities by reabsorbing or excreting bicarbonate and excreting nonvolatile acids. For example, acidosis may occur as a result of lactate production in anaerobic metabolism or ketone production in the absence of insulin. Bicarbonate can be lost with prolonged diarrhea, resulting in a relative increase in $[H^+]$ concentration. Renal failure can result in a direct increase in the accumulation of nonvolatile acids. This, of course, results in a relative decrease in the bicarbonate concentration.

▼ PHYSIOLOGICAL COMPENSATION

The body will always attempt to counterbalance an acid–base disturbance via a compensatory mechanism. For example, respiratory acidosis invokes a secondary metabolic response by increasing renal bicarbonate retention. This is an attempt to correct the acid–base balance by bringing the pH back into the normal physiological range (7.35–7.45). A metabolic acidosis invokes a secondary ventilatory response to increase ventilation and remove carbon dioxide. This mechanism results in the removal of greater quantities of volatile acids in an attempt to return pH to a more compatible physiological level.

It should be kept in mind that although there is an attempt to return pH to normal, complete compensation does not occur. This occurs in part because of the gradual decrease in stimulus as the pH gets closer to the normal value. The expected compensation for a metabolic acidosis is as follows:

$$PaCO_2 \, (\pm 2) = 1.5 \times \text{plasma bicarbonate} + 8$$

A patient with a metabolic acidosis resulting in a plasma bicarbonate of 15 mmol/L would have an expected $PaCO_2$ of

$$PaCO_2 \, (\pm 2) = 1.5 \times 15 + 8$$
$$= 30.5 \text{ mmHg} \, (\pm 2 \text{ mmHg})$$

Therefore, this metabolic acidosis should result in a $PaCO_2$ between 28.5 and 32.5 mmHg. If the $PaCO_2$ is above or below this value, compensation is abnormal and a respiratory abnormality exists. If the expected compensation does not exist, underlying respiratory abormalities are likely to exist.

Because the physiological response to a metabolic alkalosis is not consistent with an acidosis, an alternate formula for prediction is necessary. The expected $PaCO_2$ for a metabolic alkalosis can be calculated as follows:

$$\text{Expected } PaCO_2 \, (\pm 2 \text{ mmHg}) = \text{plasma bicarbonate} + 9$$

Therefore, with a plasma bicarbonate of 35 mmol/L, the expected $PaCO_2$ is

$$PaCO_2 \, (\pm 2 \text{ mmHg}) = 35 + 9$$
$$= 44 \text{ mmHg} \, (\pm 2)$$
$$= 42 - 46 \text{ mmHg}$$

Because hypoventilation results in hypoxia and general alveolar instability, it has very limited compensatory reserves for alkalosis.

Respiratory acidosis results in renal compensation through retention of bicarbonate. The expected level of compensation can be calculated by using the following formula:

$$\text{Change in bicarbonate} = [\text{Change in } PaCO_2/10] \times 2.5$$

Therefore, an increase of $PaCO_2$ to 60 mmHg from the normal value of 40 mmHg should result in the following plasma bicarbonate concentration if normal compensation is present:

$$\text{Change in bicarbonate} = [20/10] \times 2.5$$
$$= 2 \times 2.5$$
$$= 5$$

As a result, a normal plasma bicarbonate of 24 mmol/L would increase to 29 mmol/L in an attempt to return the pH back toward normal. Plasma bicarbonate seldom rises above 45 mmol/L to compensate for a respiratory acidosis.

Respiratory alkalosis or hyperventilation results in excretion of bicarbonate through the kidneys. The expected reduction in bicarbonate for a reduction of $PaCO_2$ to 20 mmHg.

$$\text{Expected change in } HCO_3^- = [20/10] \times 4$$
$$= 2 \times 4$$
$$= 8$$

Therefore, a normal plasma bicarbonate of 24 mmol/L would decrease to 16 mmol/L in an attempt to return the pH to normal. Plasma bicarbonate seldom decreases to below 12 mmol/L when responding to a respiratory alkalosis.

▼ RULES OF THUMB FOR CHANGING pH

There are rules of thumb used to estimate changes in pH. The important thing to remember about these rules is that they are designed to keep information organized and easier to remember.

In this text, the measured value of $PaCO_2$ plays a significant role in calculating pH change. The governing rule of thumb is as follows: a $PaCO_2$ change of 10 mmHg will affect the pH by 0.08 pH units (Table 14-2).

There are four metabolic indices used in North America: plasma bicarbonate, standard bicarbonate, total carbon dioxide, and BE/deficit. All four are calculated values derived from $PaCO_2$ and pH. The differences between these indices were described earlier in this chapter. Remember, there is little advantage to be gained by using more than one index. Choose one and stick with it. For the purpose of this exercise, BE/deficit will be used.

However, plasma bicarbonate can be used if you set 24 as the zero point. The mean value is zero and the range is ±2 mmol/L (meq/L) within two standard deviations. Again, zero will be considered the neutral point, and positive

TABLE 14-2	pH Changes Associated with CO_2 Changes		
pH	pH Units	$PaCO_2$	$PaCO_2$ Change
7.64	0.24	10	10 mmHg
7.56	0.16	20	10 mmHg
7.48	0.08	30	10 mmHg
7.40		40	
7.32	0.08	50	10 mmHg
7.24	0.16	60	10 mmHg
7.16	0.24	70	10 mmHg

TABLE 14-3 pH Changes Associated with Base Changes

pH	pH Units	BE/BD	HCO$_3^-$ Change
		(excess)	
7.85	0.45	+30	10 mmol/L
7.70	0.30	+20	10 mmol/L
7.55	0.15	+10	10 mmol/L
7.40	0.00	0	0
7.25	0.15	−10	10 mmol/L
7.10	0.30	−20	10 mmol/L
6.95	0.45	−30	10 mmol/L
		(deficit)	

values will be considered indicative of potential alkalosis. A negative value will be considered heading indicative of a developing acidosis (Table 14-3).

The rule of thumb used in this case will be that a base excess or deficit of 10 mmol/L (meq/L) will change the pH by 0.15 pH units.

▼ ELECTROLYTES AND METABOLIC ABNORMALITIES

Electrolytes can provide important clues about the origin of an acid–base abnormality. Because potassium is shifted extra- or intracellularly by acid–base disturbances, it is often abnormal when pH is outside the normal range. Metabolic acidosis results in hyperkalemia because the hydrogen ion exchange is with intracellular potassium or sodium. A drop in pH of 0.10 pH units can increase plasma potassium levels by as much as 0.6 mmol/L. Potassium is reduced with metabolic alkalosis. If this response is not exhibited, normal potassium homeostasis is unlikely.*

In summary:

1. High plasma potassium + low plasma bicarbonate = metabolic acidosis.
2. Low plasma potassium + high plasma bicarbonate = metabolic alkalosis.

Sodium and chloride concentrations can also be helpful when evaluating acid–base disturbances.

1. Plasma sodium concentration is affected by changes in hydration.
2. Plasma chloride is affected by hydration and hydrogen ion concentration (dehydration results in decreased sodium and chloride).

---

* This response does not always occur. If the potassium level is inappropriate, abnormal body potassium homeostasis is likely.

TABLE 14-4 Metabolic Acidosis	
Anion Gap Disorders	**Nonanion Gap Disorders**
1. Ketoacidosis	1. Diarrhea
2. Lactic acidosis	2. Carbonic anhydrase inhibitors
3. Chronic renal failure	3. Ingestion of a chloride–salicylate overdose containing acid
5. Methyl alcohol ingestion	4. Renal tubular acidosis
6. Ethylene glycol ingestion	5. Enteric drainage tubes

Therefore, if the chloride changes normally without a corresponding change in sodium, then an acid–base abnormality is likely.

Metabolic Acidosis (Anion Gap)

An anion gap is a concept used to estimate electrolyte levels by substracting the sum of chloride and bicarbonate anions from the number of sodium or potassium cations. It can be useful in the interpretation of acid–base abnormalities (Table 14-4).

$$Anion\ gap = Na^+ - (Cl^- + HCO_3^-)$$
$$= 142 - (103 - 26)$$
$$= 13$$

A normal range for the anion gap is 12–14 mmol/L. This gap results from the unmeasurable anions in the blood such as proteins and phosphates. When an ion such as lactate is produced during anaerobic metabolism, plasma bicarbonate is reduced and the gap is increased. Therefore, this simple calculation can be used to identify a metabolic acidosis (anion-gap acidosis). If chloride is elevated, the anion gap can be normal even in the face of metabolic acidosis. This is commonly referred to as a nonanionic gap acidosis or hyperchloremic acidosis.

Metabolic Alkalosis

Metabolic alkalosis is one of the most common acid–base disorders. This occurs in one of two ways: as a result of bicarbonate gain through administration or from loss of nonvolatile acids, a condition that can be reversed by nasogastric suction or blood transfusion containing citrate.

Arriving at a diagnosis of metabolic alkalosis is best accomplished by following the approach to interpretation given below.

A Step-By-Step Approach to Interpretation
1. Is the pH normal (between 7.35 and 7.45)? A pH < 7.35 is indicative of acidemia, whereas a pH > 7.45 is indicative of alkalemia.

2. Compute the anion gap if acidosis is present.
3. Is the HCO_3^- normal, elevated, or decreased appropriately?
4. Is the $PaCO_2$ normal (35–45 mmHg)? Elevated (>45 mmHg)? Reduced (<35 mmHg)? And if so, is there an appropriate ventilatory compensation?
5. Consider electrolyte variations.
6. Is oxygenation adequate?

▼ IS OXYGENATION ADEQUATE?

The answer to this question is variable depending on the clinical goal. Generally, a PaO_2 between 80 and 100 mmHg is normal. A value below 80 mmHg is indicative of hypoxemia, whereas a value above 100 mmHg indicates hyperoxia. A rule of thumb here is to attain a PaO_2 as close to the patient's normal value as possible. For a patient with chronic obstructive pulmonary disease, this may be a value below 70 mmHg. If records do not exist, a physical assessment of the patient may provide valuable clues. If the metabolic component indicates a chronic imbalance from a long-term attempt to compensate for respiratory insufficiency, the patient's normal PaO_2 is likely depressed. With carbon monoxide poisoning or procedures that might potentially affect gas exchange, hyperoxygenation and a higher PaO_2 (above 100 mmHg) are not only acceptable but necessary.

▼ MIXED VENOUS BLOOD GASES

Arterial blood gases are indicative of the oxygen supply to the tissues, telling us about oxygen demand and supply. If demand exceeds supply, which is determined by cardiac output and local perfusion for a specific area, mixed venous blood gas values will begin to deteriorate ($P\bar{v}O_2$ and $S\bar{v}O_2$ will decrease). Demand is determined by metabolic rate and is increased by disease or exercise. Mixed venous oxygen values can be a reflection of the effectiveness of the body's ability to meet gas exchange demands. Monitoring can give an early indication of developing cardiopulmonary disturbances.

The normal physiological response to hypoxemia is to increase cardiac output to increase oxygen supply. As long as cardiac output is increased, arterial and mixed venous oxygen partial pressure remain relatively unchanged as the demand is being met. If cardiac output decreases, PaO_2 can remain relatively normal, but $P\bar{v}O_2$ and $S\bar{v}O_2$ drop because supply has decreased and demand has remained the same.

TABLE 14-5	Normal Mixed Venous Blood Gas Values	
pH	7.33–7.43	(7.38)
$PvCO_2$	46–48 mmHg	(47)
PvO_2	35–45 mmHg	(40)
SvO_2	75%	

Mixed venous blood is present in the pulmonary artery (Table 14-5). A sample should be drawn for analysis through a pulmonary artery catheter, which is placed as distal as possible to ensure complete mixing of blood from all parts of the body (Figure 14-1). Analysis of this sample can yield one of the following diagnoses:

1. Severe anemia will reduce oxygen delivery or supply to the tissues, and if demand remains unchanged, the PvO_2 and SvO_2 will decrease.
2. Carbon monoxide poisoning can also severely hamper oxygen delivery to the tissues. Although PaO_2 may be relatively normal, SaO_2, PvO_2, and SvO_2 will all be decreased.
3. Septic shock results in metabolic dysfunction, hindering the cell's

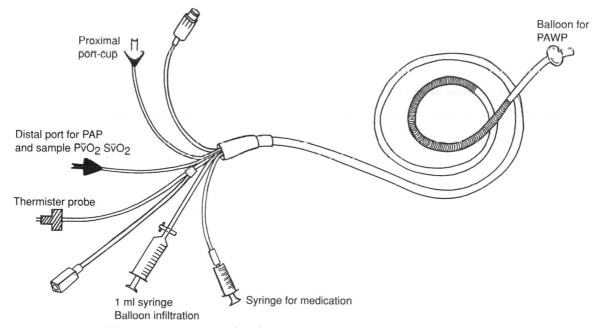

Figure 14-1.   A sample of a pulmonary artery catheter used to draw blood samples for analysis and to monitor pulmonary pressures.

TABLE 14-6.	Blood Gases							
	1	2	3	4	5	6	7	8
pH	7.40	7.32	7.48	7.46	7.25	7.30	7.60	7.35
$PaCO_2$	40	30	50	40	38	20	43	55
BE	+1	+2	+11	+4	−10	−25	+12	+5
HCO_3	25	26	35	27	14	6	36	29

Interpretation: 1, normal blood gas values; 2, respiratory alkalosis; 3, metabolic alkalosis and respiratory acidosis; 4, metabolic alkalosis; 5, metabolic acidosis (because the respiratory system normally compensates this is indicative of an abnormal respiratory component, respiratory acidosis); 6, metabolic acidosis and respiratory alkalosis; 7, metabolic alkalosis; and 8, compensated respiratory acidosis (normal pH below 7.4 with a high PCO_2).

ability to use oxygen. Blood gases may look normal, and an increased cardiac output may be present. $P\bar{v}O_2$ and $S\bar{v}O_2$ can actually be elevated in the presence of severe hypoxia.

▼ INTERPRETATION OF BLOOD GAS VALUES

The possible diagnoses related to inadequate oxygenation, as determined by abnormal blood gases, include

1. respiratory acidosis.
2. respiratory alkalosis.
3. normal $PaCO_2$.
4. metabolic acidosis.
5. metabolic alkalosis.
6. normal metabolic component.

The best way to learn how all of these components fit together is by example. For this reason, Table 14-6 provides blood gas values and shows how they are interpreted in clinical practice. It is extremely important to keep in mind that this is only one component of your clinical investigation.

Common sense combined with a systematic approach to clinical investigation is the surest way to succeed in this regard.

▼ CONCLUSION

Blood gases are an important part of evaluation in cardiopulmonary care. However, it must always be kept in mind that they are only a small part of the overall picture that must be considered during the evaluation process. One can use blood gases, in combination with other relevant clinical data, to document, quantify, and specify a disease process.

❖ Review Questions

1. The normal values for $PaCO_2$, PaO_2, and SaO_2 are
   a. 35–45, 80–100, and 98%.
   b. 20–30, 70–80, and 100%.
   c. 80–100, 30–40, and 85%.
   d. 45–50, 60–80, and 92%.
   e. 35–45, 75–80, and 95%.
2. $PaCO_2$ is measured using a
   a. Clark electrode.
   b. polarographic electrode.
   c. Severinghaus electrode.
   d. spectrophotometer.
   e. Sanz electrode.
3. Which of the following disorders may result in an anion gap acidosis?
   i. Ketacidosis
   ii. Lactic acidosis
   iii. Diarrhea
   iv. Chronic renal failure
   v. Salicylate overdose

   a. iii, iv, v
   b. ii, iii, iv
   c. i, ii, iii
   d. i, ii, iv, v
   e. i, ii, iii, iv, v

Questions 4–8: Diagnose the condition of the patient by interpreting the following blood gases:

	1	2	3	4	5
pH	7.32	7.46	7.30	7.60	7.35
$PaCO_2$	30	40	20	43	55
BE	+2	+4	−25	+12	+5
HCO_2	26	27	6	36	29

4. (Column 1)
   a. Respiratory alkalosis
   b. Metabolic alkalosis
   c. Metabolic acidosis and respiratory alkalosis
   d. Metabolic alkalosis
   e. Compensated respiratory acidosis
5. (Column 2)
   a. Respiratory alkalosis
   b. Metabolic alkalosis
   c. Metabolic acidosis
   d. Respiratory acidosis
   e. Compensated respiratory acidosis

6. (Column 3)
   a. Metabolic alkalosis and respiratory acidosis
   b. Respiratory acidosis
   c. Metabolic alkalosis
   d. Respiratory acidosis and metabolic alkalosis
   e. Metabolic acidosis and respiratory alkalosis
7. (Column 4)
   a. Respiratory acidosis and metabolic alkalosis
   b. Respiratory alkalosis
   c. Metabolic acidosis
   d. Metabolic alkalosis
   e. Respiratory acidosis
8. (Column 5)
   a. Compensated metabolic alkalosis
   b. Compensated respiratory acidosis
   c. Respiratory alkalosis
   d. Metabolic acidosis and respiratory acidosis
   e. Metabolic alkalosis

15

PULMONARY DEFENSE MECHANISMS

OBJECTIVES

1. List the functions of the nose.

2. Describe mucociliary clearance.

3. Characterize the mucus layer in the respiratory tract.

4. Discuss how mucus is produced.

Matthews LR: CARDIOPULMONARY ANATOMY AND PHYSIOLOGY. © 1996 Lippincott–Raven Publishers.

5. Contrast and compare the cough and sneeze reflexes.

6. Describe the sigh mechanism.

7. Explain how an invading insult is localized.

8. Describe nonciliated airway clearance.

9. Explain lymphatic clearance as a defense mechanism.

10. Discuss the merits of the immunological defense mechanisms.

11. Give an example of cell-mediated immunity.

12. Reiterate the lines of defense in the lung.

13. Give details on the defensive response to oxidant injury.

14. Describe the role of alpha-1 antitrypsin.

Our discussion of the lungs has assumed (unless otherwise noted) smooth inhalation uninterrupted by trauma or pathophysiology. Such a focus has necessarily relieved us of the need to examine the body's built-in pulmonary defense mechanisms, which come into play to protect the lungs against invasion by organisms and particulate matter. Because the lungs are essentially open to the environment, pollutants and organisms present in the air pose a constant threat. For this reason the lungs must have lines of defense designed to deal with organisms and particles of various sizes.

This multifaceted defense process can be broken down into six categories:

1. The nose and nasal passageways
2. Mucociliary clearance
3. High-velocity clearance and reflex responses
4. Nonciliated airway clearance
5. Lymph and blood clearance
6. Immunological defense

▼ THE NOSE

The hair in the vestibule of the nose acts as a filter that traps large particles. The change in the direction of airflow resulting from turbulence also aids **inertial impaction**, a process in which the particles become trapped and immobilized up against the mucosal wall. This matter gets removed by ciliary activity or physically blowing the nose. Particle deposition is enhanced as well by the dramatic decrease in airflow velocity that occurs once airflow passes the nares.

The mucosa has antibacterial properties, which protect the respiratory tract against the potentially infectious organisms that remain trapped in the mucous layer until they are gradually removed back into the posterior pharynx. There, they are swallowed. This system is effective for filtering out normal environmental particulate matter that is inspired through the nose, but it can be easily bypassed by mouth breathing.

Airflow Through the Nose

During nasal breathing, inspired air enters the nostrils at an angle of about 60 degrees to the floor of the nose. Approximately 2 cm beyond the entrance, the air flows past the narrowest point (ostium internum) and then bends to travel along the nasal passages. The majority of air passes the middle meatus, seldom more than 1 mm from the surface. During inspiration some air from the sinuses mixes with the nasal stream, and during expiration gas enters the sinuses. The two nasal airstreams join at the nasopharynx and bend to move vertically downward. The turbulence created by the gas flow directional changes promotes inertial impaction of any airborne particulate matter.

The nose has a built-in flow-limiting device, which is designed to collapse when flow exceeds 1 L/sec. This results from the pressure decrease created during forced inspiration. When ventilatory demands are high, we resort to mouth breathing. It is interesting to note that as airflow increases, as in exercise, resistance in the nasal passages actually decreases. However, the efficiency of the nasal passage (possibly extending to the oropharynx) as an air conditioner is significantly reduced under these circumstances.

Because nasal breathing provides superior protection against airborne intruders, it offers the best protection against environmental injury. Conversely, oropharyngeal breathing, which allows for the inspiration of larger, potentially more damaging particles, results in maximum hazard.

Particle Deposition

Deposition of inhaled particles in the nasal passages is determined by the nature of airflow and the physical characteristics of the particles themselves. The most important characteristics are gravitational settling, inertial impaction, diffusion, and interception.

Gravitational Settling
Particles fall steadily when under the influence of gravity. This influence is directly related to the size and density of the particles.

Inertial Impaction
Particles tend to travel in straight lines and impact on obstructions. When gas flow changes direction (such as at a bifurcation) or velocity (such as occurs at an opening or narrowing of an airway), particles tend to leave the airstream and impact up against the mucosa.

Diffusion

This pertains to particles less than 1 cm in diameter. Gas molecules begin to interface with the movement of these particles. At this point, diffusion from variations in concentration becomes more significant than sedimentation.

Interception

This results when the inhaled particle (i.e., a foreign body) is of sufficient size to lodge in a passageway.

Nasal Secretory Antibody

The principal secretory immunoglobulin is IgA. When antigenic stimulation occurs, rapid local synthesis of the antibody takes place to combat invading allergens.

▼ MUCOCILIARY CLEARANCE

The **mucociliary escalator** is one of the lung's primary defense mechanisms. It provides protection by trapping bacteria, particulate matter, and cellular debris in its cilia, and then sweeping it out of the conducting airways to be swallowed or coughed up.

The cilia (Figure 15-1) are bathed in a nonviscial layer of serous fluid, known as the *sol layer*. They make contact with the mucous layer on top, which

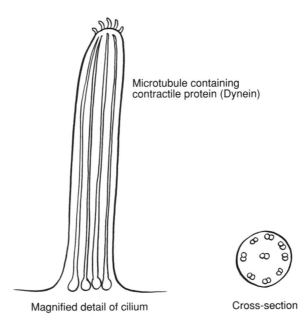

Microtubule containing
contractile protein (Dynein)

Magnified detail of cilium   Cross-section

Figure 15-1.   Magnified detail of cilium.

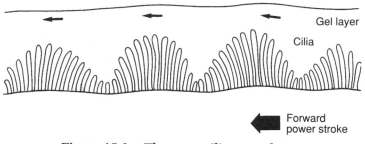

Figure 15-2. The mucociliary escalator.

is known as the *gel layer*. The cilia beat at a frequency of 11–15 beats/sec in the form of a wave that moves the mucous layer progressively up the airway. It actually has an easy backward stroke and a forward stroke in the direction of the larynx. A contractile protein known as dynein is responsible for the ciliary movement. This moves mucus at a velocity of about 1 cm/min, removing trapped particles up and out of the airways (Figure 15-2).

Mucus

Lining the respiratory tract is the aqueous mucus layer, which is approximately 10–20 μm thick and consists of the sol and gel layers. Respiratory tract mucus consists of approximately 95% water and 5% particulate matter. The particulate matter includes 2–3% protein and glycoproteins, 1% lipids, and 1% minerals. The proteins include immunoglobulins and alpha-1 antitrypsin (a bacterial enzyme inhibitor). Glycoproteins (compounds made up of a carbohydrate and a protein) are most responsible for the gelatinous nature of airway secretions. It is estimated that approximately 10–100 mL of mucus is produced per day in the normal healthy lung. Close attention to proper systemic hydration is important in both health and disease.

It is the function of the mucus lining to trap invasive organisms and particles before they can make their way into the vulnerable lungs. The smaller the particle, the farther into the respiratory tract it can travel before becoming trapped and then expelled. Particle sizes greater than 30 μm deposit in the mouth, larynx, and trachea. Particles of 3–10 μm deposit on the mucus layer along the bronchial tree. Particle of 1–3 μm can reach the alveolar regions. Once deposited, the mucociliary escalator transports the particle up and out to be swallowed or coughed up.

Production of Secretions

Respiratory lining secretions are produced by a number of different cells and glands: goblet cells, submucosal glands, myoepithelial cells, Clara cells, and serous cells (Figure 15-3).

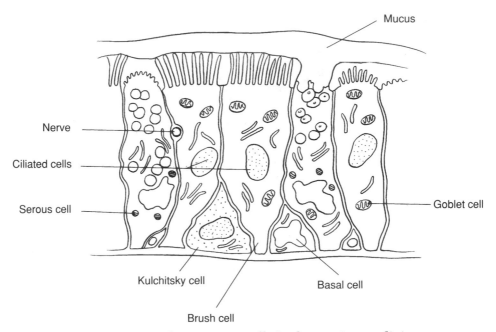

Figure 15-3. The secretory cells in the respiratory lining.

Goblet Cells

These mucus-producing cells, which are stimulated primarily by irritation, produce a glycoprotein that contributes to the mucus blanket.

Submucosal Glands

Found in the tracheobronchial tree, these glands are the major contributors to mucus found in the respiratory tract. Each submucosal gland consists of a ciliated duct and a collecting duct, as well as mucus tubules and serous tubules.

Each substructure has a specific function that plays a role in defending the airways from invasion by organisms and particles.

The ciliated duct connects with the airway wall and is itself lined with cilia, just as the airway is. The collecting duct is a nonciliated tube about 1 mm in length that abruptly turns into a secretory (mucus) tubule.

Mucus tubules are branches that arise from the collecting duct and attach to the serous tubules. The serous tubules arise from the surface of the ductlike little "buds." The serous secretions must pass over the mucus and both secretions then pass into the collecting duct.

From the collecting duct, secretions pass into the ciliated duct and then on into the airway lumen.

Myoepithelial Cells

These cells are located beneath the serous, mucus, and collecting duct cells. They contain fibrils that can contract and promote the passage of secretions along the secretory tubules and a collecting duct that then conveys the secretions out into the airway.

Clara Cells

These nonciliated cells are found peripherally, mostly in the terminal bronchioles. Although these cells do secrete a fluid, it is different from the secretions produced by the goblet and serous cells. The purpose of Clara cell secretions is still unknown.

Serous Cells

These cells are found outside the mucous glands and are more centrally located than Clara cells. Irritation, drugs, and infection can all increase the number of Clara and serous cells. This may also result in a conversion of these cells to mucous cells.

▼ HIGH-VELOCITY CLEARANCE AND REFLEX MECHANISMS

The Cough Reflex

The cough is initiated by a reflex that is initially stimulated by any foreign matter or irritation of the bronchi or trachea. The larynx and carina are particularly sensitive to touch, and the terminal bronchioles and alveoli are sensitive to irritating corrosive chemical stimuli such as chlorine gas.

Afferent impulses enter the medulla through the vagus nerves and cause the following chain of events:

1. A deep breath, usually over 2 L in volume, is taken.
2. The epiglottis closes and the vocal cords also shut.
3. The abdominal muscles contract and push up on the diaphragm, increasing intrathoracic pressure to over 100 cm H_2O.
4. The epiglottis and vocal cords open suddenly, expelling gas and free particles out of the bronchi and trachea.

The Sneeze Reflex

The sneeze is initiated by a reflex that is triggered when any foreign matter or irritation is detected in the nasal passageways. The afferent impulses pass through the fifth cranial nerve to the medulla. The reflex is essentially the same as the cough reflex except that the uvula is depressed and a large portion of air passes quickly through the nose. This is an attempt to remove the foreign material from the nasal passages.

The Sigh Mechanism

Approximately 12–15 times per hour, we take a deep breath. In some cases it approaches maximum inspiratory capacity. This reflex is tied to the maintenance of the functional residual capacity and is extremely important to continuous mucociliary clearance (see Chapter 5).

▼ NEURONAL INVOLVEMENT

The body always attempts to localize an invading insult. Constricting the airways and increasing airway secretions are just two of the mechanisms designed to accomplish this task.

The lungs are innervated by the autonomic nervous system, the part of the nervous system responsible for controlling involuntary functions. Afferent fibers from the stretch, cough, and irritant receptors travel through the pulmonary plexus to the vagus nerve (Figure 15-4). Receptors from the nose and nasal sinuses enter the central nervous system through the trigeminal and glossopharyngeal nerves.

All parasympathetic efferent fibers are contained in the vagus nerve. These fibers carry motor impulses to the smooth muscle and glands of the tracheobronchial tree. Stimulation of these nerves results in increased bronchial smooth muscle tone (bronchoconstriction), glandular secretion, and vasodilation.

Sympathetic efferents arise from the T1, T2, T5, and T6 to enter the sym-

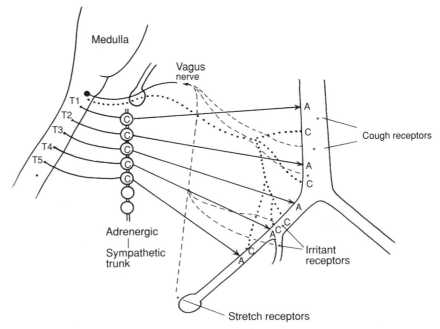

Figure 15-4. Neuronal involvement.

pathetic trunk and the pulmonary plexus. Generally, this stimulation results in bronchodilation and decreased mucus secretion.

▼ NONCILIATED AIRWAY CLEARANCE

Clearance out of the peripheral lung is slow in comparison with clearance from lung regions lined with cilia. This region is the alveolar surface, and primary mechanism of clearance is by alveolar macrophage. (Macrophages are the major phagocytes in the immune system, whose function is to identify and ingest foreign matter.) These alveolar macrophages are part of the mononuclear phagocyte system. Large numbers of tissue macrophages are a part of the alveolar walls. Particles entrapped in the alveoli can be phagocytized, digested, and released into the lymphatics or encapsulated in an attempt to limit their impact. These cells are actively motile and have the ability to clean up the alveolar surface after it has been covered by foreign bodies.

▼ BLOOD AND LYMPH CLEARANCE

Because large molecule pulmonary invaders cannot move across the epithelium for inactivation, they must be taken care of by alternate means. Some substances are eliminated by absorption into the blood. Solid substances can be absorbed by the bronchial lymphoid tissue, which is particularly responsive to chronic irritation. In fact, this tissue seems to become more extensive when irritated.

Vascular Response to Inflammation

The immediate response to injury or invasion is momentary constriction of the small vessels in the invaded area. This response is followed immediately by vasodilation of both the arterioles and venules responsible for supplying the area. This hyperemia is accompanied by an increase in capillary permeability and allows fluid to escape into the tissue, resulting in edema. This exudate helps dilute the toxic or irritating agent. Eventually, white blood cells (WBCs) accumulate in the area, and blood flow stagnates and clots, which aids in the localization of the injury.

Lymphoid Response

In the thymus (a gland situated in the mediastinum anterior to and above the heart), epithelial cells produce soluble factors important in the maturation of lymphocytes. This process takes about 2–3 days, after which the mature lymphocytes (thymic lymphoid or T cells) move from the thymus gland into the bloodstream. From there, lymphocytes enter the inner cortex of the lymph nodes, spleen, and other lymphoid tissue, from which they can most efficiently perform their role in the cellular immune response to systemic invasion.

Lymph Nodes

Lymph nodes serve to (1) remove foreign material from lymph before it enters the bloodstream and (2) act as centers to proliferate immune cells.

Because lymph nodes are spongelike structures, macrophages, lymphocytes, and granulocytes move slowly through them. This meshwork provides a surface for macrophages to attach to and phagocytose antigens (Figure 15-5).

▼ IMMUNOLOGICAL DEFENSES

The invasion of the respiratory tract provides considerable opportunity for the body to mount a defensive response. B-lymphocytes are lymphoid stem cells that originate in the bone marrow and then migrate to the spleen and lymph nodes, where they are responsible for humoral immunity. Humoral immunity results in the elimination of bacterial invaders, neutralization of bacterial toxins, prevention of viral reinfection, and immediate allergic responses. B-cell clones produce different types of immunoglobulins and provide them with the specificity necessary to react to a single antigen.

Respiratory immunoglobulins play an important role in the defense of the respiratory tract. IgG, IgM, IgE, and IgA are all produced by cells in the lungs and upper respiratory tract. IgG and IgM are produced in regional lymph nodes, and IgE is produced in lymph tissue of the upper respiratory tract. IgA is formed in the regional nodes and the mucosal lining. Elevated levels of IgE are indicative of an allergic response resulting from contact with an antigen. The airways also contain clear cells, which are involved in defense, probably as immunoblasts. (Table 15-1 lists specific immunoglobulins and their characteristics.)

TABLE 15-1   Immunoglobulins: Their Abundance and Characteristics

Class	Abundance	Characteristics
IgG	75%	Exists in most B cells; contains antiviral, antitoxin, and antibacterial antibodies; crosses the placenta; responsible for protection of newborn; activates complement and binds to macrophages
IgA	15%	Exists primarily in body secretions, such as saliva, nasal and respiratory secretions, breast milk; protects mucous membranes
IgM	10%	Forms the natural antibodies such as those for ABO blood antigens; important in early immune response; activates complement
IgD	0.2%	Little is known of its action but may affect B-cell maturation
IgE	0.004%	Binds to mast cells (these cells synthesize and store histamine) and basophils (type of WBC); involved in allergic and hypersensitivity reactions; elevated serum levels in extrinsic asthma

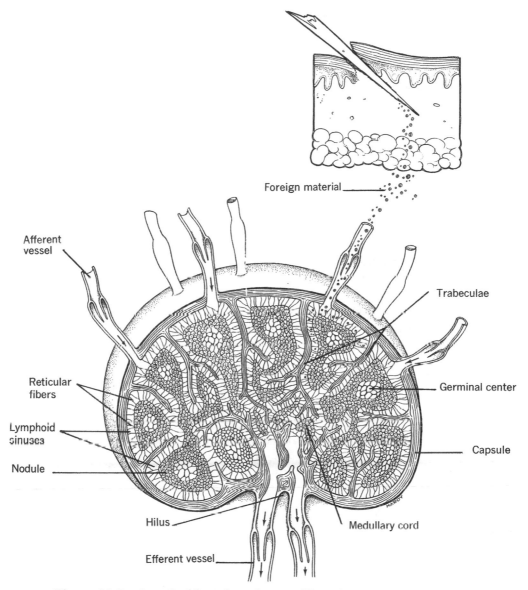

Figure 15-5.   A typical lymph node as it filters foreign material from the lymph fluid. (Chaffee, E.E. and Lytle, I.M., Basic Physiology and Anatomy, 4th ed. Philadelphia: J.B. Lippincott, 1980, with permission.)

Cell-Mediated Immunity

This form of immunity involves an interaction between the circulating macrophage and the T-lymphocyte (T cell). T-lymphocytes are sensitized to a specific antigen, then begin to release a protein called lymphokinase, which is responsible for sensitizing more T cells to increase macrophage activity in the affected area. Chemical mediators also bring more lymphocytes into the area. The T cells produce a cytotoxic effect necessary to protect against intracellular pathogens such as *Pneumocystis carinii* and other viruses.

Cellular Response to Inflammation

The cellular response to acute inflammation involves

1. margination of WBCs.
2. emigration of WBCs.
3. chemotaxis.
4. phagocytosis.

Margination of White Blood Cells

As fluid leaves the capillaries, blood viscosity increases. When this happens, leukocytes begin to marginate, or move to the periphery of the blood vessel and adhere to the vessel lining. The term *pavementing* describes the cobblestone appearance on the vessel lining.

Emigration of White Blood Cells

This is the mechanism by which the leukocytes extend pseudopods (false feet), which enable them to pass through the capillary wall by ameboid movement. They then migrate into the tissue spaces by a process known as **diapedesis**. Red blood cells (RBCs) also emigrate into the tissue. Interstitial osmotic pressure is increased by this process, and fluid follows these cells, causing edema.

Chemotaxis

Once through the cell wall, leukocytes move through the tissue space guided by the presence of bacterial and cellular debris, for which they have a particular attraction. This ability of cellular debris and bacteria to attract additional WBCs to the site of inflammation is known as **chemotaxis**, which can be either positive or negative.

Phagocytosis

The final response involves engulfing and degrading bacterial and cellular debris, a process known as **phagocytosis**. Neutrophils, the most common granulocytic WBCs, are at times referred to as microphages because they phagocytose bacteria and small particles. Monocytes may be called macrophages because they remove tissue debris and larger particles.

In summary, the lungs' primary lines of defense against invasion become

TABLE 15-2   Lines of Defense

First Line: Mechanical Barrier

Sneeze
Cough
Mucociliary escalator
Secretory immune system

Second Line: Phagocytosis

Monocytes
Lymphocytes
Macropohages

Third Line: Immune System

B-lymphocytes (immunoglobulins)
T-lymphocytes
Secretory immunity

increasingly more complex as they change from purely mechanical processes such as the sneeze to the intricate processes of immune system response (Table 15-2).

▼ OTHER PROTECTIVE MECHANISMS

Response to Oxidant Injury

The alveolar capillary membrane can be damaged by inhaled noxious agents. This can occur when pollutants such as ozone are inhaled or when above normal levels of oxygen are breathed. Type 1 pneumocytes are most susceptible to this form of injury. Type 2 cells proliferate in an attempt to repair the damage and replace the nonfunctional Type 1 cells. This process results in a lung that is more tolerant of insults of this type.

Inhaling oxidants into the lung results in peroxidation of unsaturated lipids in cellular membranes, which eventually results in visible tissue damage. Antioxidants such as alpha tocopherol (vitamin E) or hydroxy compounds can increase the tolerance level also. Gradual increases in oxygen concentrations may result in an acquired tolerance because of an increased capacity to maintain glutathione in the reduced state. This is accomplished by the presence of nicotinamide-adenine dinucleotide phosphate (NADPH), an enzyme found following exposure to oxidants. Glutathione is known to be an important antioxidant in RBCs and phagocytes.

Alpha-1 Antitrypsin

Alpha-1 antitrypsin appears to be important in the neutralization of proteases, enzymes that break down the peptide bonds that hold amino acids together as proteins and that are released by lysed leukocytes involved in the defense process. The ongoing structural integrity of lung elastin and collagen depends on this antienzyme. Normal serum levels of alpha-1 antitrypsin are between 2 and 4 g/mL. Lower than normal levels are associated with panlobular emphysema.

▼ CONCLUSION

The lungs are very vulnerable organs that are, in many respects, at the mercy of airborne bacteria and particulate matter. To minimize the risk posed by these potential invaders, the body came up with a series of pulmonary defense mechanisms. These mechanisms range from the mechanical (as exemplified by sneezing or coughing) to the physiologically more sophisticated systems of immunological defenses and antienzyme activity. These lines of defense give the body an array of possibilities for filtering out and/or inactivating invasive organisms so that the seemingly effortless work of spontaneous ventilation can be carried out without interruption.

❖ Review Questions

1. The aqueous mucus layer lining the respiratory tract
   i.   is 10–20 μm thick.
   ii. traps mucus smaller than 1 μm.
   iii. consists of the sol and gel layers.
   iv. contains 10% protein, 5% lipids, and 1% mineral.
   v.   moves at a velocity of about 1 cm/min.

   a. i, ii, iv
   b. iii, iv, v
   c. i, iii, iv
   d. i, iii, iv, v
   e. All of the above

2. Which of the following immunoglobulins is contained primarily in body secretions?
   a. IgA
   b. IgG
   c. IgM
   d. IgD
   e. IgE

3. The cellular response to acute inflammation involves
   i.   the margination of WBCs.
   ii. emigration of WBCs.
   iii. chemotaxis.
   iv. phagocytosis.

   a. i, ii, iii

    b. ii, iii, iv

    c. i, ii, iv

    d. i, iii, iv

    e. i, ii, iii, iv

4. Phagocytosis is

    a. engulfing and degrading bacterial and cellular debris.

    b. leukocyte movement through the tissue space guided by the presence of bacteria.

    c. leukocyte extension of pseudopods for passage through the cell wall.

    d. T-lymphocyte production of cytotoxins.

    e. part of the complement system's response to an autosomal crisis.

Bibliography

American Heart Association. *Textbook of Advanced Cardiac Life Support.* 1994.

Barnes TA. *Respiratory Care Principles: A Programmed Guide to Entry-Level Practice,* 3rd ed. Philadelphia: F.A. Davis Company, 1991.

Branson RD, Hess DR, Chatburn RL. *Respiratory Care Equipment.* Philadelphia: J.B. Lippincott Company, 1995.

Burton GC, Hodgkin JE, Ward JJ. *Respiratory Care: A Guide to Clinical Practice,* 3rd ed. J.B. Lippincott Company, 1991.

Des Jardins T. *Cardiopulmonary Anatomy and Physiology: Essentials for Respiratory Care,* 2nd ed. Albany, NY: Delmar Publishers Inc., 1993.

Des Jardins T. *Clinical Manifestations of Respiratory Disease,* 2nd ed. Chicago: Year Book Medical Publishers, Inc., 1990.

Guyton AC. *Textbook of Medical Physiology,* 7th ed. Philadelphia: W.B. Saunders Company, 1986.

Hodgkin JE, Connors GL, Bell CW. *Pulmonary Rehabilitation: Guidelines to Success,* 2nd ed. J.B. Lippincott Company, 1993.

Kacmarek RM, Mack CW, Dimas S. *The Essentials of Respiratory Care,* 3rd ed. St. Louis: Mosby-Year Book, Inc., 1990.

Loach J, Thomson, NB, Jr. *Hemodynamic Monitoring,* J.B. Lippincott Company, 1987.

Miller WF, Scacci R, Gast LR. *Laboratory Evaluation of Pulmonary Function.* J.B. Lippincott Company, 1987.

Rose BD. *Clinical Physiology of Acid Base and Electrolyte Disorders.* New York. McGraw-Hill Book Company, 1977.

Shapiro BA, Kacmarek, RM, Cane RD, Peruzzi WT, Hauptman D. *Clinical Application of Respiratory Care,* 4th ed. St Louis: Mosby-Year Book Inc., 1991.

West JB. *Pulmonary Pathophysiology—the Essentials,* 4th ed. Baltimore: Williams & Wilkins, 1992.

West JB, *Respiratory Physiology—the Essentials,* 5th ed. Baltimore: Williams & Wilkins, 1995.

Wilkins RL, Sheldon RL, Krider SJ. *Clinical Assessment in Respiratory Care,* 2nd ed. St. Louis: The C.V. Mosby Company, 1990.

Matthews LR: CARDIOPULMONARY ANATOMY AND PHYSIOLOGY. © 1996 Lippincott–Raven Publishers.

Glossary

Acidemia A lower than normal pH in arterial blood; a higher than normal [H^+] concentration (pH < 7.35).

Acidosis A state in which there is a lower than normal base. There may or may not be an accompanying acidemia.

Active transport Transport that requires energy; these processes must be linked to energy metabolism or expenditure in some way.

Acute respiratory failure Failure of any of the components involved in oxygen transport or use to meet the metabolic demands of the body.

Acute ventilatory failure A condition in which the respiratory pump does not maintain carbon dioxide homeostasis without metabolic compensation.

Afterload The pressure encountered by the contracting ventricle.

Alkalemia A higher than normal pH in arterial blood; a lower than normal [H^+] concentration (pH > 7.45).

Alkalosis A state in which there is higher than normal base. There may or may not be an accompanying alkalemia.

Alveolar deadspace The volume of inspired gas that reaches an alveolus but does not participate in gas exchange.

Alveolar ventilation The portion of ventilation that exchanges gas molecules with pulmonary blood; effective ventilation; respiratory rate times tidal volume less the physiologic deadspace ($RR \times V_T - V_D$).

Anatomical deadspace The total volume of gases contained in the airways from the mouth or nose down to the alveoli.

Anatomical shunt Blood that passes from right to left in the heart without traversing the pulmonary capillaries (thebesian, bronchial, and pleural circulation).

Anemia A deficiency of red blood cells (RBCs) caused by (1) rapid blood loss, (2) aplastic anemia, (3) megaloblastic anemia, or (4) hemolytic anemia. *Microcytic hypochromic anemia* is a condition caused by rapid blood loss in which RBCs produce insufficient hemoglobin. *Aplastic anemia* is a lack of RBCs resulting from insufficiently functioning bone marrow and is often caused by radiation or chemical poisoning. *Megaloblastic anemia* results from a deficiency in one of the factors responsible for the production of erythroblasts in the bone marrow. *Hemolytic anemia* is a hereditary condition, characterized by fragile RBCs that rupture easily.

Anion gap The difference between measured cations and anions; ($Na^+ + K^+$) $- (Cl^- + HCO^{3-}$); the normal range is 15–20.

Anoxia Absence or total lack of molecular oxygen.

Apnea Cessation or absence of breathing movement.

Matthews LR: CARDIOPULMONARY ANATOMY AND PHYSIOLOGY. © 1996 Lippincott–Raven Publishers.

Apneusis Sustained inspiration.

Asphyxia A condition of restricted or even absent gas exchange.

Baroreceptor A specialized neural structure that senses changes of system arterial or venous pressure and reflexively initiates compensatory changes of heart rate and systemic vascular resistance.

Bohr effect The effect of CO_2 or H^+ on hemoglobin's affinity for oxygen (i.e., CO_2 causes decreased hemoglobin's affinity for O_2).

Bronchial breath sounds Normal tracheal and main bronchial sounds. Expiration is higher pitched and more intense than that heard with vesicular breath sounds. Bronchial breath sounds heard over distal lung areas are abnormal and indicative of consolidation.

Bronchodilator tone The state of contraction or relaxation of smooth muscle in the bronchial walls that regulates airway caliber.

Capillary shunt Perfusion in the absence of ventilation.

Cardiac asthma Bronchospasm resulting from pulmonary edema.

Cardiogenic shock Failure to maintain blood supply to the circulatory system and tissues because of inadequate cardiac output.

Catabolism The processes by which complex substances are converted to simpler substances, usually with the release of energy.

Central venous pressure The pressure in the right atrium.

Chemotaxis Movement of additional white blood cells to an area of inflammation in response to chemical mediators.

Chronic respiratory failure Chronic inability of any of the components involved in oxygen transport or use to meet the metabolic demands of the body.

Chronic ventilatory failure A chronic condition in which the lungs are unable to maintain carbon dioxide homeostasis with metabolic compensation or near normal pH.

Compliance The measurement of distensibility; the inverse of elastance; a change in volume divided by a change in pressure.

Conductance Opposite of resistance, or the tendency to conduct.

Conjugated protein A protein containing protein molecules as well as other molecules.

Crackles Rales; crackling breath sounds (similar to crushing cellophane), usually heard on inspiration, produced as a result of fluid in small- to medium-sized airways.

Cyanosis A bluish-purple discoloration that first becomes apparent when the concentration of deoxyhemoglobin (reduce) in the capillary blood of the skin, mucous membranes, or nail beds exceeds 5 g/dL.

Deadspace The total volume of all non–gas-exchanging or conducting airways in the lung. Any space in the respiratory system that receives inspired gas and does not participate in gas exchange.

Diapedesis The passage of blood cells through the unruptured wall of a capillary vessel.

Dicrotic notch Indicates aortic closure and is visible during arterial blood pressure monitoring on the downstroke of the waveform.

Diffusing capacity (DL) The rate of gas transfer through a permeable membrane. Units for pulmonary diffusing capacity are mL/min/mmHg.

Diffusion atelectasis The collapse of gas exchange units (alumsli) resulting from the diffusion of gas out of the unit into the blood in response to a diffusion gradient. May be associated with high oxygen concentration or static ventilation.

Diffusion block A disease process that reduces diffusion of gases across the A/C membrane by changing the diffusion characteristics of the membrane.

Dynamic A condition of changing volume; hence, flow is not zero.

Dynamic compliance A measure of the maximum airway pressure (peak) required to deliver a given V_T (minus PEEP).

Dyspnea Difficult or labored breathing.

Edema A swelling of the brain caused by a build-up of fluid, a result of trauma that disrupts the pressure balance of fluid movement between the capillary bed and the interstitium.

Elastance The inverse of compliance, a static pressure change divided by a change in volume.

Eupnea Normal comfortable breathing at rest.

Expiratory reserve volume The maximum amount of volume of gas that can be exhaled after the end of a normal spontaneous expiration.

Flail chest Multiple rib fractures involving more than two ribs broken in two or more places, resulting in paradoxical chest movement.

Functional residual capacity The amount of air remaining in the lungs at the end of a normal expiration.

Glycogenesis The conversion of lactic acid, glycerol, and pyruvic acid to glucose and then to glycogen.

Haldane effect The effect of oxygen saturation on hemoglobin's affinity for CO_2.

Hamburger phenomenon The chloride shift that occurs in the red blood cell.

Hematocrit Percentage of volume of packed red blood cells.

Hemodynamics The forces involved in circulating blood through the body.

Hemoglobin The iron-containing pigment of red blood cells, which carry oxygen and carbon dioxide to and from the tissues of the body. Abnormal forms of hemoglobin are due to mutations. *Hemoglobin A* is adult hemoglobin, which contains two α and two β polypeptide chains. *Hemoglobin A_2* is a variation of hemoglobin A, containing two α and two γ polypeptide chains. *Hemoglobin F* is fetal hemoglobin, which contains two α and two γ polypeptide chains.

Hemolysis The destruction of red blood cells, resulting in an insufficient number of cells available for gas transport.

Histotoxic hypoxia A condition in which cellular hypoxia exists due to cellular inability to use available oxygen.

Hypercapnia Abnormally high carbon dioxide pressure within a biological system.

Hypercarbia (or hypercapnia) An elevated arterial carbon dioxide tension.

Hyperoxia Increased or abnormally high oxygen concentration or pressure within a biological system.

Hyperpnea Increased breathing frequency and/or tidal volume.

Hyperventilation Pulmonary ventilation rate or volume that exceeds the metabolic requirements of the body. Best identified by the affect it has on arterial carbon dioxide levels ($PaCO_2 < 30$ mmHg).

Hypocapnia (also called hypocarbia) A reduced arterial carbon dioxide tension (below 35 mmHg).

Hypopnea Decreased breathing frequency and/or tidal volume compared with breathing at rest.

Hypotension The reduction in systolic and diastolic pressure.

Hypoventilation Pulmonary ventilation rate that does not meet the metabolic demands ($PaCO_2 > 50$ mmHg).

Hypoxemia A reduced blood oxygen tension ($PaO_2 < 80$ mmHg in adults).

Hypoxemic hypoxia A condition in which hypoxia is caused by arterial blood that has a lower than normal tension.

Hypoxia A term implying inadequate tissue or cellular oxygenation. Circulatory, or stagnant, hypoxia is an insufficient blood supply causing a reduction in transported gases.

Hysteresis The difference between the respiratory and expiratory flow curves.

Ineffective circulating volume A volume of blood that bypasses the capillary circulation through an arteriovenous fistula (shunt).

Inertial impaction The removal of a particle from suspension because of its initial tendency to go in a straight line and impact on the wall of an airway.

Inspiratory capacity The maximum volume of a gas that can be inhaled after normal exhalation of a tidal volume.

Inspiratory reserve volume The maximum volume of a gas that can be inhaled after the end of a normal spontaneous inspiration.

Intrapleural pressure The pressure within the lung; this term is synonymous with intrathoracic pressure.

Intrapulmonary pressure The pressure within the lung; this term is synonymous with static airway pressure and is usually expressed as an average.

Methemoglobin The heme molecule in its normal, ferrous state.

Minute volume The number of breaths per minute multiplied by tidal volume ($RR \times V_T$).

Mixed venous blood A mixture of venous blood from all parts of the body. In practice, blood taken from the pulmonary artery.

Mucociliary escalator The mucus blanket of the airways in intact beating cilia that is responsible for continuously cleansing the lungs of embedded particulate matter.

Muller's maneuver Inspiratory effort against a closed airway or glottis.

Obstructive alterations An increase in overall lung volume.

Orthopnea Difficulty in breathing in the recumbent position, especially the supine position, which is relieved by sitting or standing.

$P(A-a)O_2$ Alveolar to arterial oxygen tension gradient; the difference between the oxygen tension in the alveolus (PAO_2) and the oxygen tension in arterial blood (PaO_2); $PAO_2 - PaO_2$.

Paradoxical movement A movement that is contrary to the normal function of a system (chest moves in instead of out).

Passive diffusion Movement of a substance through a membrane that requires only a concentration gradient. No energy is required.

Phagocytosis The ingestion and digestion of bacteria and particles by phagocytes.

Physiological deadspace The portion of ventilation that does not exchange with the alveolar unit; the sum of anatomical and alveolar deadspace.

Physiological shunt The total percentage of cardiac output that does not exchange gas with alveolar air (total venous admixture).

Pickwickian syndrome Obesity–hypoventilation syndrome.

Pleural effusion The failure of fluid reabsorption caused by an increase in colloidal osmotic pressure, which is a result of infection.

Pneumothorax The presence of air or gas outside the lungs but still inside the thorax.

Preload This term refers to the degree of stretch of the myocardium at the moment before it contracts.

Pulse pressure The difference between systolic and diastolic pressures.

Rebreathing The breathing of exhaled gases.

Residual volume The volume of a gas remaining in the lungs after a maximum expiration.

Resistance The difficulty encountered while moving a flow of gas through an airway.

Respiratory alternans A paradoxical chest movement resulting from alternating diaphragm and intercostal breathing.

Respiratory exchange ratio The ratio of carbon dioxide production per unit time to oxygen consumption per unit time across the alveolar capillary membrane.

Respiratory insufficiency Altered function of the lungs producing clinical symptoms, usually including dyspnea.

Respiratory quotient The ratio of carbon dioxide production per unit time to oxygen consumption per unit time at a cellular level.

Respiratory rate The number of breaths per minute.

Resistance The difficulty encountered while moving a flow of gas through narrow or constricted airways.

Restrictive alteration A reduction in overall lung volumes.

Rhonchi Coarse breath sounds heard during expiration and resulting from secretions in the larger airways.

Shunt A vascular communication that bypasses normal circulatory channels. A *right-to-left shunt* refers to blood that leaves the right side of the heart and enters the left side of the heart without entering the pulmonary circulation or passing a ventilated alveolus. Also known as intrapulmonary shunting.

Shunt effect Due to perfusion in excess of ventilation.

Spontaneous ventilation Breathing; the process by which oxygen from the external environment is taken into the lungs, exchanged for carbon dioxide, and then released into the environment.

Stasis atelectasis The collapse of gas exchange units resulting from static lung volumes (low V_T and high RR) in the absence of a sigh. Commonly associated with inactivity, postoperative pain, or any process that results in a reduction in thoracic movement.

Static compliance A measure of compliance using the airway pressure required to hold the lungs and chest wall at end inspiration when gas flow is not present.

Stridor An inspiratory breath sound audible to the unaided ear. The sound is produced by a large airway obstruction.

Stroke work The work required for the left and right ventricles to raise the blood pressure during each contraction.

Tachypnea Rapid breathing that is characterized by an increased frequency, even at rest.

Thalessemia A group of hereditary conditions resulting in a defect in the synthesis of one or more of the polypeptide chains of hemoglobin, which cause failure of or decrease in the synthesis of the affected chain. α Thalessemia is characterized by impaired synthesis of the α chain; β thalessemia is a reduction or absence of the β chain.

Tidal breathing Consecutive breaths characteristic of spontaneous ventilation.

Tidal volume The volume of gas inspired and expired with each breath.

Transairway pressure The pressure difference between mouth and alveolar pressure.

Transpulmonary pressure The difference between alveolar and intrapleural pressure; alveolar pressure minus intrapleural pressure.

True shunt (also called absolute shunt) That portion of venous blood that in some way finds its way from the right side of the heart (venous blood) to the left side of the heart for distribution to the body and does not take part in gas exchange in the lungs.

Valsalva maneuver Expiratory effort against a closed glottis or airway.

Venous admixture Composed of a mixture of venous and arterial blood.

Ventilation-perfusion ($\dot{V}/\dot{Q}$) ratio The ratio of alveolar ventilation to capillary blood flow.

Vesicular breath sound Normal parenchymal sounds, which are accentuated during inspiration. In abnormal conditions, a localized decrease or absence of sound may be present.

Vital capacity The maximum volume of gas that can be exhaled after the deepest possible inspiration.

Wheezing The high-pitched, whistling breath sound heard during expiration; produced by bronchospasm and present in bronchospastic disorders.

Appendix 1:
ABBREVIATIONS AND SYMBOLS

a—arterial blood
A—alveolar gas
ABG—arterial blood gas
ADH—antidiuretic hormone
A/E—air entry with auscultation
AG—anion gap
AP—anterior/posterior
ARDS—adult respiratory distress syndrome
ASD—atrial septal defect
ATP—adenosine triphosphate
ATPD—ambient temperature and pressure dry
ATPS—ambient temperature and pressure saturated
AV—atrioventricular

B—barometric
BE—base excess
BMR—basal metabolic rate
BP—blood pressure
BPM—breaths per minute
BSA—body surface area
BTPS—body temperature and pressure saturated

c—capillary
C—content (mL/dL or mL/L)
CaO_2—oxygen content of arterial blood
$C(a-\bar{v})O_2$ — arterial to venous oxygen content difference
CBC—complete blood count
CcO_2—oxygen content of capillary blood (also CiO_2)
CF—cystic fibrosis
CHF—congestive heart failure
cm H_2O—centimeters of water pressure
CNS—central nervous system
CO—carbon monoxide
CO_2—carbon dioxide
CoHb—carboxyhemoglobin
COPD—chronic obstructive pulmonary disease
CPR—cardiopulmonary resuscitation

Matthews LR: CARDIOPULMONARY ANATOMY AND PHYSIOLOGY. © 1996 Lippincott–Raven Publishers.

CSF—cerebrospinal fluid
Cst—static compliance
$C\bar{v}O_2$—oxygen content of mixed venous blood
CVP—central venous pressure

DL—diffusing capacity
DL_{CO}—diffusing capacity of carbon monoxide
DPG—diphosphoglycerate

ECG—electrocardiogram
ERV—expiratory reserve volume
$ETCO_2$—end-tidal carbon dioxide

$FEF_{25\text{-}75}$—forced expiratory flow rate at 25% and 75% of vital capacity (MMEFR)
$F_{ET}CO_2$—fractional exhaled end-tidal CO_2
$F_{\bar{E}}CO_2$—fractional mixed exhaled CO_2
FEV_1—forced expiratory volume per second
FEV_1/FVC—ratio of exhaled volume at 1 second to forced vital capacity expressed as a percentage
FIO_2—fractional inspired oxygen concentration expressed as a decimal
FRC—functional residual capacity
FVC—forced vital capacity

Hb—hemoglobin
HbCO—carboxyhemoglobin
$HbCO_2$ — carbaminohemoglobin
HbF—fetal hemoglobin
Hbmet—methemoglobin
HbO_2—oxyhemoglobin
HCO_3^-—bicarbonate
Hct—hematocrit
He—helium
HR—heart rate

IC—inspiratory capacity
ICP—intracranial pressure
IRV—inspiratory reserve volume

L—liter
L/min—liter(s) per minute
LVEDP—left ventricular end-diastolic pressure
LVH—left ventricular hypertrophy
LVSW—left ventricular stroke work

max—maximum
MetHb—methemoglobin
MMEFR—maximal mid-expiratory flow rate
mmHg—millimeters of mercury pressure (torr)
MAP—mean arterial pressure

O_2—oxygen

PA—posterior/anterior
P_A—alveolar pressure
$P(A\text{-}a)O_2$ — alveolar to arterial oxygen gradient expressed in mmHg
PAC—premature atrial contraction
$PaCO_2$ — partial pressure of carbon dioxide in arterial blood
$P_{alveolar}$—alveolar pressure
PAP—pulmonary artery pressure
$\overline{PAP}$—mean pulmonary artery pressure
PAT—paroxysmal atrial tachycardia
Paw—airway pressure (proximal)
$\overline{Paw}$—mean airway pressure
PAWP—pulmonary arterial wedge pressure
P_B — barometric pressure
$P_{\bar{E}}CO_2$ — partial pressure of mixed exhaled carbon dioxide
PEFR—peak expiratory flow rate
$P_{ET}CO_2$ — partial pressure of end-tidal carbon dioxide
PFT—pulmonary function testing
PIP—peak inspiratory pressure
PVC—premature ventricular contraction
$P\bar{v}CO_2$ — partial pressure of carbon dioxide in mixed venous blood
$P\bar{v}O_2$—partial pressure of oxygen in mixed venous blood
PVR—pulmonary vascular resistance
PVRI—pulmonary vascular resistance index

$\dot{Q}_S$—shunted cardiac output
$\dot{Q}_t$—total cardiac output
$\dot{Q}_S/\dot{Q}_t$—shunted cardiac output ratio

R—resistance
R_{AW}—airway resistance
RBC—red blood cell
RQ—respiratory quotient
RR—respiratory rate
RV—residual volume
RVH—right ventricular hypertrophy
RV/TLC—ratio of residual volume to total lung capacity

SaO_2—arterial oxygen saturation
S_pO_2—oxygen saturation by pulse oximetry

STPD—standard conditons: temperature 0°C, pressure 760 mmHg, and dry (0 water vapor)

SVC—slow vital capacity

$S\bar{v}O_2$ — mixed venous oxygen saturation

SVR—systemic vascular resistance

SVRI—systemic vascular resistance index

$TcPO_2$—transcutaneous oxygen

T_E—expiratory time

T_I—inspiratory time

T_{ID}—dynamic inspiratory time

T_{IS}—static inpiratory time

TLC—total lung capacity

v—venous

$\dot{V}$ —flow

$\dot{V}_D$—ventilation per minute of physiologic deadspace

$\dot{V}_A$—minute alveolar ventilation

VC—vital capacity

$\dot{V}CO_2$—carbon dioxide production (STPD)

V_D—deadspace

V_E—minute volume or expired volume per minute (BTPS)

$\bar{v}$—mixed venous

$\dot{V}_{max50}$—maximum flow rate at 50% of volume

$\dot{V}_{O2}$—oxygen consumption

$\dot{V}/\dot{Q}$—ventilation/perfusion ratio

VSD—ventricular septal defect

V_T—tidal volume

V_{TDel}—delivered tidal volume

V_{TG}—thoracic gas volume

$\bar{x}$—bar above any symbol indicates a mean value

$\dot{x}$—dot above any symbol indicates a time derivative

Appendix 2:
GAS SYMBOLS AND LAWS

▼ GAS SYMBOLS

Gas	Symbol
Carbon dioxide	CO_2
Ethylene	C_2H_4
Helium	He
Nitrogen	N_2
Nitrous oxide	N_2O
Oxygen	O_2
Oxygen–carbon dioxide mixtures	$O_2\text{-}CO_2$
Oxygen–helium mixtures	$O_2\text{-}He$

▼ GAS LAWS

Boyle's law states that when temperature and the amount of a gas remain constant, pressure and volume vary inversely:

$$P_1V_1 = P_2V_2$$

Charles' law states that when pressure and the amount of a gas remain constant, the temperature and volume of a gas will vary directly:

$$V_1/T_1 = V_2/T_2$$

Gay-Lussac's law states that when volume and the amount of a gas remain constant, the pressure and temperature of the gas vary directly:

$$P_1/T_1 = P_2/T_2$$

Fick's law states that the rate of gas diffusion across a membrane is directly proportional to the surface area of the membrane (A), to the diffusion constants of the membrane (D), and to the difference in partial pressure of the gas between the two sides of the membrane ($P_1 - P_2$), and is inversely proportional to the thickness of the membrane (T):

$$\dot{V} \text{ gas } \alpha \, [A.D. \, (P_1 - P_2)]/T$$

Matthews LR: CARDIOPULMONARY ANATOMY AND PHYSIOLOGY. © 1996 Lippincott–Raven Publishers.

Graham's law states that the rate of diffusion of a gas is directly proportional to the solubility coefficient of the gas and inversely proportional to the square root of the gram molecular weight (GMV) of the gas:

$$\frac{\text{Diffusion rate for } CO_2 = \sqrt{\text{GMW } O_2} = 32}{\text{Diffusion rate for } O_2 = \sqrt{\text{GMW } CO_2} = 34}$$

Henry's law states that the amount of gas dissolved in a liquid (ΔC) at a given temperature is proportional to the partial pressure of the gas (ΔP):

$$\Delta C = \alpha \Delta P$$

where α is the solubility coefficient of gas in liquid.

Ideal gas law states that

$$PV = nRT \text{ or } R = PV/nT$$

Answers to Review Questions

CHAPTER 1:

1. a
2. a
3. d
4. d
5. c
6. c
7. a

CHAPTER 2:

1. c
2. b
3. b

CHAPTER 3:

1. b
2. a
3. b
4. e
5. e
6. c
7. e
8. a
9. c

CHAPTER 4:

1. a
2. d
3. c
4. c
5. e
6. d
7. a
8. d
9. c
10. a

CHAPTER 5:

1. d
2. b
3. e
4. a
5. b
6. a
7. c

CHAPTER 6:

1. c
2. a
3. c
4. c
5. b
6. c
7. b
8. d
9. d
10. a
11. e
12. a
13. e

CHAPTER 7:

1. b
2. d
3. c
4. a
5. e
6. c
7. e
8. d
9. c
10. b
11. c
12. c

CHAPTER 8:

1. c
2. b
3. c
4. d
5. c

CHAPTER 9:

1. c
2. a
3. d
4. d
5. d
6. a
7. c
8. a
9. c
10. e

CHAPTER 10:

1. c
2. a
3. d
4. e
5. a
6. c
7. a
8. c
9. d
10. b

CHAPTER 11:

1. a
2. c
3. e
4. e
5. b
6. c
7. e
8. a
9. c
10. a

CHAPTER 12:

1. e
2. d
3. c
4. c
5. e
6. d

CHAPTER 13:

1. a
2. e
3. c
4. b
5. d
6. a

CHAPTER 14:

1. a
2. c
3. d
4. a
5. b
6. e
7. d
8. b

CHAPTER 15:

1. c
2. b
3. e
4. a

Index